Candle[lights]

FOR THE WORLD

Transforming the World Through Deeds of Kindness

Candlelights for the Family

CAREGIVER'S WORLD

Spiritual Keys for Avoiding Caregiver Burnout and Promoting Inner Peace

By Alice W. Johnson, Ed.D.
In Collaboration with husband, John Johnson, Jr., Ed. D.

authors of

Mysterious Stranger Aboard
Love Paints Beauty in the Soul
Let Your Attitude Be Gratitude
The Calm and the Strife
Symbols of Love
Love Finds Expression Through Kindness and Concern
Caring for the Caregiver
We Create Our Own Happiness

Published by Mal-Jonal Productions, Inc., Miami, Florida

Mal-Jonal Productions, Inc.,
16713 SW 107th Place
Miami, Florida 33157-2965

Printed in the United States of America

Library of Congress Cataloging-in-Publication Data
Johnson, Alice and John
Candlelights for The Family Caregiver's World:
How to Avoid Caregiver-Burnout
and Promote Inner Peace

ISBN 0-9715031-0-9

Contents

Acknowledgements

When we were told by our psychologist that writing is good therapy, and he counseled us to write through the pain of our suffering triggered by the debilitating disease of multiple sclerosis, my husband and I went on a writing spree.

Thanks to Dr. Jack W. Kensinger, our psychologist, for his professional counseling that enabled us to successfully adjust to the world of family caregiving, and for awakening us to the surprise that we are creative writers. Thanks to Dr. John T. McAdory, our family physician, for professional health care throughout the writing spree.

Thanks to talk show hostess Oprah Winfrey for steering our writing into the spiritual world of gratitude journaling that awakened us to transcendent wisdom and universal compassion, and for girding our flight into authoring a Candlelights series.

An overwhelming thanks to our outstanding "America's Caregiver and Candlelight," President George W. Bush, for his dynamic leadership in guiding us through the shocking pain of the September 11, 2001, terrorists attacks on America, and for counseling us to be strong and courageously continue with our lives in building this great USA with our myriad of talents. Adhering to his wise counseling, we dried our tears and, using our healing therapy, began writing this book...the beginning of a Candlelights series designed to touch lives and lift spirits.

Many, many thanks to our wonderful parents for raising us in a spiritual home atmosphere. We will always feel the love of their family caregiving and kindness.

Thanks to our teachers, ministers, counselors, friends, co-workers; and to my sorority, Delta Sigma Theta, Inc., for the many deeds of kindness that have enriched our lives.

A special thanks to John Penney, our graphic artist, for preparing our book for publication; to Janell Walden Agyeman of Marie Brown Associates for guiding our writings with wisdom, insight and encouragement and to our manuscript readers, Edith Oden and Delores Washington for long hours of intensive reading.

We especially thank the Miami, Florida Veterans Administration Medical Center professional caregiving staff and resident patients for further extending our insights into the Kingdom of God where my husband and I saw universal love and kindness in action, and where we learned that all creation is holy, even our adversities.

Compassionately dedicated to the world of family caregivers and their disabled loved ones.

Introduction

Then shall the righteous answer him, saying, "Master,
when did we ever see you hungry, or thirsty,
or a stranger, or naked, or sick, or in prison
and did not help you?" And he will answer,
"When you did it to these my brothers
you were doing it to me."
—Matthew 25:37-40

Prelude

Praying silently from the depths of her soul and humbly serving as a voice for other family caregivers, the weary traveler asked, "Kind Master, why are there so many sick, disabled and suffering people in this world?"

The Master softly answered, "They are here to teach you kindness and compassion, my child, so that you can be a candlelight for the world."

1. Focusing The Spiritual Mission

Yes, our disabled brothers are here to teach us how to cultivate kindness and compassion toward one another because kindness is the true religion. Family caregiving is a spiritual mission designed to teach this basic universal truth, guiding us humbly into pathways of vision and showing us the face of God. Thus enroute, we experience the voyage, the victor and the victory.

The wisdom of family caregiving teaches us that pain and death are inevitable, but suffering is a choice. For this reason, caregivers need to know how to avoid the stressful suffering that comes from long-term caregiving and how to find inner peace.

The National Family Caregivers Association (NFCA) reports that family caregivers (the people who care for disabled family members or friends) experience sadness, frustrations and clinical depressions more than the rest of the population. The NFCA also finds that the needs of family caregivers are distinct from the needs of those for whom they care, and that three-fourths of all family caregivers are women. Many of these women are victims of "caregiver-burnout" and are crying out for help.

"Baby Boomers," that segment of the population who now are reaching 50 years old, are likely to spend more years caring for their elderly parents than they did raising their own children. They face a most complicated challenge they never prepared for inasmuch as many elderly will live to age 100 and beyond.

2. *Need for the Book*

Because family caregivers share a common bond despite the differences in their individual situations, I, in collaboration with my husband, John, who has multiple sclerosis...a disease of the central nervous system that robs motor skills...decided to write this book. In our 45-year battle as caregiver and recipient, we have found some effective coping strategies that have been most helpful to us in mastering stress to avoid "caregiver-burnout", to live a meaningful and productive life, and to enjoy inner peace.

During our research and while attentively following the suggestion of talk show hostess Oprah Winfrey to engage in gratitude journal writing, we learned that:

(1) More family caregivers become critically ill and enter nursing homes because of caregiver-burnout, rather than due to an exacerbation of their own physical condition.

(2) Many caregivers experience clinical depression with suicidal and homicidal tendencies because of caregiver-burnout. They simply cannot handle the tremendous physical, emotional and other demands of their responsibilities.

(3) Family caregiving is a gift of miracles...a brilliant **candlelight** that leads the caregiver to the metaphysical world of the spirit in which he joyfully sees the face of God and falls to his knees in humility and gratitude. When he can truly see caregiving in this light, he does not ask, "Why me?" but "Why not me?" His spirit of humility becomes a candlelight for gratitude journal writing, lighting up his world and the world of those around him. God (Love) is the light within him. Gratitude journal writing is the key that unlocks that light.

(4) Gratitude journal writing is the key to the family caregiver's inner life. It is a form of meditation that enhances growth and constitutes the greatest source of spiritual support imaginable. It is a pathway to the soul that awakens the spirit to its inherited divinity and the joy of spreading love and compassion.

(5) Gratitude journaling is spiritual psychotherapy, a learning institution that testifies to the gift of caregiving, if family caregivers would but utilize it. It is a life-saving, life-altering activity that yields "fruits of the spirit" for family caregivers.

(6) Gratitude journal writing is the epitome of personally communicating with God. It is the ultimate path of "Writing to Him" who lives within us, and listening humbly and meditatively to the sound of His silent voice as He answers

the soul's attitude with the wisdom He has already placed within us. We share with humanity this direct line of creation by "Writing for Him," using our gift of writing as a ministry to serve and fulfill Him.

"Be humble before God, yet great in Him."

3. Attitude is Everything

My husband's and my ninth book of gratitude journaling under the motif: "Writing For Him," and entitled *Candlelights for the Family Caregiver's World*, is drawn from the lessons of our undaunted, 45-year battle with a debilitating, presently incurable disease. It humbly whispers through the pages of our journals, "Lord, order my steps in Your Word." Gratitude journaling revealed to us that within us all are the answers of creation.

On the journey, we have learned that attitude is everything. We have learned that cultivating an attitude of gratitude in the spirit of kindness and compassion is excellent holistic medicine for the mind, body and soul.

Through gratitude journal writing, we have found that the lessons drawn from our human experiences have enabled us to view caregiving as a spiritual mission in which the caregiver is called to be a candlelight for Eternal God. Knowing that there is no light more brighter than *His* light of love that shines within us, we found joy in answering the call. We answered the call with a passion, making it a religious vocation, a ministry. We now understand what clergymen once told us: "Our vocation is a direct line of creation, from God through us to all mankind. We must be humble before God, yet great in Him."

Our counselors taught us that a vocation is a perceived call or invitation from God to accomplish a certain work or live out one's life in a certain way. With this insight, we learned to accept caregiving as a vocation...a gift of opportunities granted the caregiver to obey the will of Eternal God by spreading love and kindness.

We have different gifts...If it is contributing to the needs of others, let us give generously. —Romans 12:6-8.

In gratitude for this spiritual gift and in a bond of compassion for those who care for disabled family members or friends, we joyfully share spiritual keys that may be used as a mini-course in caring for the family caregiver. It is our hope that these keys will help abate caregiver-burnout and promote inner peace for the family caregiver and the care recipient, strengthening them to continue spreading "kindness and compassion" throughout the world, in obedience to the Creator's will.

By following the essential tools as outlined in *The Power of Focus*, written by Canfield, Hansen and Hewitt, we were guided to discover and live our purpose. In so doing, we were able to see clearly our need to write this book and to make a contribution to humanity. Our priority focus is to share our insight of the spiritual mission of family caregiving. The joy of loving and serving in this endeavor to help other family caregivers avoid caregiver-burnout and promote inner peace "energizes us" and gives us the high we all seek...discovering and living our purpose to help heal the world as we heal ourselves.

Spiritual Key # 1

"Writing for Him"

"...And He said unto me, 'Write, for these words are true and faithful.'" —Revelations 21: 5

WEEK ONE
Managing the Stress of Family Caregiving

Come unto me all ye that labour and are heavy laden, and I will give you rest. — Matthew 11:29

SUNDAY, Week I
Prelude

In search for inner peace and prosperity, the weary traveler prayed humbly, "Kind Master, You said that my disabled brother is here to teach me how to be a candlelight for the world. Please tell me how can he teach me wisdom for managing this stress so that I can do Your Divine Will of caring for him, even when the burdens of this world become too heavy?"

The Master replied with love and compassion, "He will teach you through your caregiving experiences how to manage the stress, my child. And he will offer strategies you will need to accomplish maximum well-being so that you can enjoy an abundant and more rewarding life and be a blessing to humanity. Through caregiving experiences, he will teach you this truth: that all things in creation are holy. But first, my child, you must be still and silently listen to the wisdom of your body, mind and spirit."

1. The Human Experience

Protecting your health must be your highest priority.
— National Family Caregivers Association

As a family caregiver, you are enduring unusual stress that can be very depressing and cause a myriad of life-threatening illnesses that are sometimes fatal, especially heart disease, which is triggered by stress.

Heart disease is today's Number One killer of women. Every minute of every day a woman dies of heart disease in the United States. It kills more women than all cancers combined, yet too often neither women nor their doctors take the threat seriously.

The National Family Caregivers Association stated in a recent report that three-fourths of all family caregivers are women, and that caregivers put so much emphasis on their care recipients' health that they neglect their own.

As a family caregiver, protecting your health must be your highest priority. Fortunately, there are ways in which you can manage the stress and take control.

Be aware that people become depressed when they isolate themselves from things that in the past have given them pleasure and joy. Try not to isolate yourself from experiences that you enjoy, especially experiences of participating in activities that promote your well being, your talents, your moral and spiritual growth.

While it is true that caregivers live with anticipatory grief in the atmosphere of death, it is very important to understand and accept the truism that: "Nobody and not anything belong to us, except in memory." Therefore, try not to be grieved by what is lost or be controlled by desire. We must all face the inevitable sorrows of life such as: the loss of all things we hold dear and the aging, sickness, and death that come to every human being.

2. Change Our Perceptions

To combat stress and replace it with feelings of contentment and inner peace, we need to change our perceptions. By changing our perceptions, we change our world.

We can do this by cultivating four common traits: high self-esteem, a feeling of personal control, a sense of optimism, and an extroverted personality. Gratitude journal writing reveals that a troubled mind cannot understand these common traits, but our continuous writing will help us eventually achieve a life of inner and outer balance.

People who feign self-esteem, soon begin feeling it.

Those who pretend to be optimistic become so.

So, if we want to combat stress and be joyful, act joyful. Even if we have to force ourselves to feel the joy. Remember, gratitude is the mother of joy. So, we must try to cultivate the joy of feeling grateful throughout the day. When we see this attitude of gratitude as a lifetime commitment and an assured stress buster that gives us inner peace, we will enjoy a balanced inner and outer life.

Follow-Up Activity:

Writing is good therapy. It is creative visualization, a program of "writing for Him" because He dwells within each of us, and within us are all the answers. His spirit is the light within you. Your body is the candle.

Find a quiet space and light a candle. Sit silently for a moment and stare into the flame. (Note: At times, throughout this mini-workshop, you might find it more convenient to light an imaginary candle when you are mediating at your workplace).

Meditate for at least five minutes, then get a notebook and silently begin a gratitude journal by focusing in on your thoughts, feelings and actions and recording them. Try to write for at least one hour or more every day. Late evenings are preferable for most caregivers. I usually write at 2 AM by candlelight, following a period of meditation, because my thoughts are clear and I am yet in communication with the Creator. Remembering my spirit, I begin "Writing for Him" who dwells within me and who has planted all the answers within me. Gratitude journaling brings them to surface and the writing becomes spontaneous.

Listening to the quiet voice within you, list five or more human experiences that are creating stress in your life today. These may include the worries and the sadness that you face every day or a shock that recently happened. Remember, gratitude journaling enables you to communicate with your soul...your higher self, and it is an excellent stress buster that can help you take control of your life, lift your spirit, and transform your world.

Try to see the stressful experiences as a divine message inasmuch as God speaks to us through everyday human experiences.

In gratitude journal writing, try to express gratitude for the experiences of being a caregiver and ask the Creator to help you see more clearly the spiritual message He is trying to convey to you so that you can adhere to it, make your daily life a blessing to others and enter into His peace.

MONDAY, Week I

Take my yoke upon you, and learn of me; for I am meek and lowly in heart: and ye shall find rest unto your souls. — Matthew 11:29

Beginning today, as you confront excessive stress, keep before you always the spiritual image of the joy you want to experience. See it, feel it, live it, love it. Develop in your mind the mood of already having a spirit of joy, then act from this viewpoint. In addition, remember to utilize the following hints as stress busters.

- Take control of your time. Set reasonable goals for you and your loved one.

- Act joyful. It can make you that way. Laugh with your loved one and others.
- Seek work that engages your skills. People are happiest when absorbed.
- Join the movement. Exercise regularly.
- Get rest. Sleep, meditate, doze.
- Give priority to close relationships. Say "I love you" to someone.
- Care for your soul. Religious people are happier.
- Remember, kindness is the true religion. Cultivate kindness toward yourself and others.

1. Cultivating the Mind

As earlier stated, a stressful, troubled mind cannot understand the wisdom that comes from gratitude journal writing. Journaling reveals that your worst enemy cannot harm you as much as your own ungrateful thoughts, feelings and actions. When these three emotions can be mastered through gratitude journal writing, no one can help you as much as your personal journaling, not even your father or your mother. In journaling, you are writing for Him who dwells within you...your higher self. He reveals to you that we are what we think, and that all that we are arises with our thoughts. When we act or speak with a negative attitude, trouble will follow us. On the other hand, when we act or speak with an attitude of gratitude, all that we are arises with our thoughts and we experience happiness.

Follow-Up Activity:

Turn the key of gratitude journal writing to open the lock to your thoughts, feelings and actions regarding today's reading. Sit quietly in the room of your higher self and try to cultivate an attitude of gratitude toward today's reading and follow-up. Try to see this as a candlelight, an opportunity for continued good health, spiritual growth, outer balance and inner peace.

TUESDAY, Week I

When pressures are released, all that is best in us has a chance to take over. —Anonymous

Stress kills prosperity; relaxation builds it. Caregivers need to experience prosperity in all areas of their tedious new world of work.

One of the ways of managing stress is cultivating the art of sitting loose and/or meditating.

You can grow out of the inner attitudes of fear, nervousness, tension and pressure which are aggravating an already existing feeling of "caregiver-burnout". The extreme experience of "caregiver-burnout" shows you the relationship between your mental and emotional attitudes and the condition of your body. When you relate the state of your mind to the condition of your experiences, you can heal yourself of the stress that is blocking the flow of the natural forces of life that cooperates with the inner consciousness.

Sitting loose and meditating can help develop those attitudes and states of consciousness which will free the natural inner forces that make for health, happiness, abundance, and freedom in your life. You can be healed from any condition by changing your inner state of mind. The effects will not disappear until the cause is removed. Your thoughts always precede your actions and reactions.

Relaxation is the starting point for managing stress.

Follow-Up Activity:
Light your candle. Today, use your keys and unlock your gratitude journal writing world. Write down five or more ways in which you can develop the art of sitting loose to combat your excessive stress. You may begin by writing: "I can develop the art of sitting loose to combat my excessive stress by saying 'Thank You' for the gift of life, health, human experiences that enhance my spiritual growth for loved ones, friends, myself," etc. Record them in your gratitude journal and try to practice feeling the love and gratitude within you, using the experience as a candlelight for continued spiritual growth.

WEDNESDAY, Week I

Relaxation is the first step in changing for the better.
It stems from understanding yourself.

Research tells us that the muscle groups around the head, face, neck, and shoulders are particularly important areas of stress that can be detrimental to your health, especially if you are a family caregiver. While it is true that a great deal of tension may accumulate in these muscles, we know that every person and/or caregiver is different. Oftentimes individuals experience tensions in the arms, hands, chest, back, stomach, hips, knees, legs, and feet while assisting with lifting a disabled loved one. It is important to be aware of what muscles seem to stay tense. It is also important to be aware that after it tenses, a muscle automatically relaxes.

Practice the habit of observing how you sit and stand in different places and at different times, especially when you are performing caregiving duties that require lifting. Try to find out which of your muscles seem to stay tense.

To manage caregiver stress, it is also important to know the difference between muscle tension and muscle relaxation. Relaxation means doing nothing with your muscles. When we practice building relaxation into everyday living, we can better manage stress and build control over the body's tension.

Follow-Up Activity:

For today, light your candle, then unlock your gratitude world and list five ways in which you can begin building relaxation into your everyday living. For example, you can build relaxation into your everyday living by:

• Meditating with feelings of thankfulness for all the negative things that could have happened but did not happen to you today.

• Meditating for a few minutes at work, or in a quiet park, recreational center, or library; while waiting in the elevator, driving your car to and from work, waiting at a red light, sitting in an office, clutching the telephone, waiting for an appointment.

Remember, always prioritize your health by practicing relaxation until it is as automatic as breathing, so that you can better help yourself and your disabled loved one.

THURSDAY, Week I

Exercise and nutrition are important in the prevention of illness and the enhancement of health.

Regular exercise and proper nutrition are stress busters because they have both physiological and psychological benefits. They are essential in combating the wear and tear of stress that results in caregiver burnout.

Regular exercise for the caregiver and care recipient

gives both a greater ability to concentrate, a reduced risk of heart attack, healthy energy, a more firm appearance, reduced anxiety and hostility, elevated mood, improved immune response, refreshing sleep, and effective control of body weight.

Do you know that we are not overweight because of what we eat? We are overweight because of why we eat. Stress is basically the "why" of our habits of overeating. Being overweight adds to our feelings of depression. To understand our attitude of depression, we need to ask ourselves: "Am I overweight because I'm depressed or am I depressed because I'm overweight?"

When you are tempted to overeat, remember that nothing tastes better than healthy "THIN" feels.

According to medical research, it is almost impossible to successfully lose weight without being officially monitored. One reason for joining such groups as Weight Watchers International is that it encourages a lifetime commitment to proper diet and exercise monitoring. The experiences Weight Watchers International recommends are "stress busters" that enable one to feel good about one's self.

Follow-Up Activity:

For today, light your candle, then grab your survival keys and unlock your gratitude journal to record your thoughts, feelings and actions about today's lesson. Record your attitude of gratitude for the wisdom of your body and your alertness to listen to it intelligently. Find out how you can begin a program of health-walking and health-eating. Record your commitment in your gratitude journal and be determined to stick with your exercise and healthy eating plan. Even a few minutes of good body stretching, walking and deep breathing periods everyday are wonderful exercises for the family caregiver. If you cannot easily get out of your home to do this, find a television fitness show and attempt to work out with the leader.

FRIDAY, Week I

Exercise releases chemicals in your body that can help relieve symptoms of anxiety and depression

We are the sum of our physical, mental and social activities. In order to enjoy good health, we need to make it a priority that these areas are being properly exercised.

Exercise helps us physically to manage stress because it relaxes the muscles.
Exercise helps vitamins fight off diseases.
Exercise can be self-enhancing and improves our responses to physical, social and mental stressors.
Exercise can be used to unclutter the mind when we walk, jog or swim.

When the body image is a stressor, whether we are overweight, too flabby, or not as muscular as we would like to be, the basic fact is that we are unhappy with ourselves. Exercise is the greatest response. People who begin an exercise program find that their self-image improves and they get an emotional lift that helps to manage stress.

When we are in good physical condition we have a greater capacity to resist excessive stress and depression. With appropriate exercise, the heart becomes more powerful and more efficient.

Follow-Up Activities:

Light your candle. Write about your attitude toward exercise. Remember to write from the heart. Try to sweep away the cobwebs and step boldly into the soul of your higher self, writing down what you are actually feeling. You are trying to change your nonchalant attitude about exercising to one of gratitude for the ability to move those muscles and joints! While it is true that we care for our bodies yet in many ways they care for themselves, we damage them with excessive stress and unnecessary weight. See your body as a special gift that needs to be exercised in order to keep it functioning properly and to abate the stress. Feel the love, respect and appreciation for your body. Record your progress in your gratitude journal.

SATURDAY, Week 1

The key to personal success is self-awareness and actualization. An individual is considered physically fit if he has stamina, suppleness, and strength. —J. Kensinger

Caregivers should be aware of the following ten characteristics of stress management which emphasize mental, physical and social health. Such awareness will curtail excessive depression.

1. Positive self-control: being well-organized in making things happen for yourself.
2. Positive self-awareness: knowing where you are going and why.
3. Positive self-esteem: feeling good about yourself.
4. Positive self-motivation: desiring to and knowing you can achieve.

5. Positive self-expectancy: deciding to excel your own abilities.
6. Positive self-image: being aware of yourself growing and changing.
7. Positive self-projection: seeing your personality and loving it.
8. Positive self-discipline: feeling mentally alert.
9. Positive self-direction: creating organized program planning.
10. Positive self-dimension: feeling good about yourself.

Gratitude journaling will reveal to you that we are great souls embodied in magnificent physical forms who are endowed with powers, talents, aptitudes and proclivities beyond our wildest dreams. In his book, The *Confessions*, St. Augustine implied that men go forth to wonder at the massive heights of mountains, the courses of the sun, moon and stars, the huge waves of the sea, the broad flow and vast compass of the rivers and oceans; and they pass by themselves without wondering at all.

We need to develop a passion for writing in our gratitude journals practically every day because this technique enables us to find our true selves. Recording our thoughts, feelings and actions will flow easily and the wisdom from the higher self will send its light into our human experiences exposing our hidden talents.

In managing the excessive stress of caregiving, life will teach us this truth: that all things in creation are holy, even the ugly, violent and incomprehensible.

Follow-Up Activities:

Light your candle. Then list five or more mental health characteristics which you would like to cultivate in order to strengthen your skills in stress management. Record your thoughts and feelings in your gratitude journal. Remember, your aim is to rid yourself of stress through gratitude journal writing and experience inner peace. When the mind is present in the heart, we call it happiness. In gratitude journaling, the mind is present in the heart because you are in communion with your soul when you pursue this silent, solitary effort.

WEEK TWO
Mastering the Art of Meditation

Let the words of my mouth and the meditation of my heart be acceptable in thy sight, O Lord, my strength and my redeemer. —Psalm 19:14.

SUNDAY, Week II
Prelude

Then the awakening traveler asked, "Kind Master, You said that my disabled brother is here to teach me how to be a candlelight for the world. Please tell me how can he teach me how to find peace within my confused and troubled mind while I am busy caring for him?"

The Master answered with love and compassion, "My child, by caring for your disabled brother, you will learn from your caregiving experiences how to master the art of meditation. Enrobed in his illness, he will teach you that meditation is the key to inner life, abundance and peace. But you must be still and quietly listen."

Meditation is the Key to Inner Life and Peace

Meditation is good for all of us, and especially the long term family caregiver who has so often experienced a world of pain and sadness. It is a precious and valuable gift of serenity that enriches the soul. A few minutes of silence do us more good than almost any other form of activity. By sitting quietly and meditating, we can relax the mind, body and spirit and experience the blessing of peace.

Peace is the gift of God's love. Meditation is a way of slowing down and getting in touch with the calm space within us. By using deep breathing and concentration techniques, a few minutes of silent meditation can help us fully relax both mentally and physically.

Meditating brings about a feeling of well-being, and helps us to get connected to the spiritual part of ourselves. The mystery is in the activity of sitting quietly and breathing deeply...inhaling and exhaling in patterns of eight seconds each for at least ten minutes to the rhythm of our personal and secret mantra. A mantra is a word sound with a special meaning. It is used in silence while inhaling and exhaling.

Research has found that people who often meditate have the need to visit their doctor far less often than those who do not. Meditation is a source of strength because it is religious and it is mind/body (holistic) medicine. Spiritual principles and faith in something greater than man can be major sources of strength for daily living and times of crisis. Meditation is a key to holistic healing.

Our minds and bodies are one. Thoughts and feelings influence our health. Emotions transfer into chemicals in our bodies. By meditating, we can collaborate with our bodies to encourage healing.

Meditation quiets your mind, allowing it to empty all of its contents either by focusing on something such as a sound, or your breathing or an idea. Meditation can be a form of imaginary gratitude journal writing. You can tell the mind what thoughts, feelings and actions your higher self would like to focus on and it will take you to the "upper room." The mind is well organized as being a good follower. You can tell the mind to focus on your breathing so that you can get beyond the conscious mind where there is some quietness. Every spiritual tradition has had a meditation tradition. Gratitude journaling is a unique spiritual tradition because it helps define you. "You" are your religion.

Meditation can help us move quietly into our feelings of stress or pain and to notice the mind's reactions, and to let go of these reactions. And then we find that there is an inner stillness and peace within some of the most difficult life situations. We learn, through meditation, that the mind has a life of its own. We human beings have a capacity for awareness and self observation. Thus, meditation is about cultivating and developing the capacity to pay attention from moment to moment. Meditation is an inner science in which we can, metaphysically and with practice, become familiar with the workings of our own bodies.

Follow-Up Activity:

First, light your candle; then begin writing down your thoughts and feelings about the importance of meditation. Include meditation on your daily agenda and try to spend at least five minutes or more a day to cultivate it. Later, if you steadfastly work to enlarge the meditation experience, then you may someday feel the joy of spending literally hours in meditation. Remember, "in silence we hear His voice" and can get clarification of situations or answers to problems.

MONDAY, Week II

Give ear to my words, O Lord, consider my meditation.
Psalm 5:1

Because silent prayer is the ultimate form of meditation, we caregivers need to master the art of meditating and make it the most important activity in our world. In meditating, we communicate with the inherited divinity within us that guides our actions, thoughts and feelings.

Genius is born in solitude. Wisdom teaches us that good conversation enriches the understanding, but solitude, a way of returning to the self, is the school of genius. When we explore the connection between solitude and the creative personality, we find that uniformity of a work denotes the hand of a single artist. Such geniuses as Beethoven, Henry James, Kipling, Shakespeare are artists who were all alone in crucial periods of their lives.

However, it is not only the outstanding people who benefit from meditation and solitude. Many ordinary people, like family caregivers, make use of meditation and solitude in times of bereavement and depression, in escaping from the pressures of daily life, in communicating with a higher power through prayer, and in finding and expressing their deepest selves. This is why gratitude journal writing is known to be an important source of man's inner happiness and psychic wholeness. It allows us to find and express our deepest selves. When we find our deepest selves, we find our creativeness. If we have a passion for our creativeness, we have the tools to be geniuses in our work. Genius is 99% passion (hard work) and merely 1% skill!

There are three stages of consciousness to consider when cultivating the art of meditation. They are called concentration, meditation, and contemplation.

To cultivate the art of concentration, we must focus on one thing. It could be the flame of a lighted candle. When we have concentrated on the flame long enough, the second stage of meditation should naturally happen. During the second stage, we move beyond the sounds of our conscious mind, forgetting everyday concerns and anxieties. Silent thoughts drift softly and slowly, and we begin receiving communications from our subconscious mind.

If we are fortunate, we enter the third stage which is called contemplation. At this stage (which could take years of practice to reach), conscious thoughts do not cross our minds and we are in touch with the pattern of the whole universe. Our spirits blend into the spirit of the universe, and we feel at home in the heart of all creation. In gratitude journal writing, we can experience how gratitude connects us to spirit, enabling us to remain in soulful silence and write deeply amid inner peace and tranquility.

Follow-Up Activity:

Again, light your candle. Continue to practice the art of meditation. Sitting firmly in a chair, practice breathing naturally and from the lower part of the lungs as you strengthen your concentration power. In your gratitude journal, write about your experience and listen closely to your thoughts and feelings.

TUESDAY, Week II

It is in the silence of the heart that God speaks to us.
— Mother Teresa

Transcendental Meditation is another form of meditation the caregiver can cultivate. It allows the mind to transcend the physical limitations of the body. People repeat a mantra over and over to help them to become more aware of what they are focusing on.

A mantra is a word or sound usually with a special meaning. In Transcendental Meditation you chant or repeat the mantra silently to yourself, concentrating on its meaning and your inner self at the same time.

The mantra is believed to wake up the three parts of our being and move us beyond the physical and into the spiritual level.

To imagine a mantra, you may:

(1) Sit quietly and comfortably, and try to relax your mind.

(2) Think of a word that you especially like.
(3) Silently repeat the word over and over, concentrating on it.
(4) Empty your mind of all other thoughts until you feel in a peaceful state. Then, you may use the word as your secret mantra when you meditate.
(5) Focus on the breathing. Breathe deeply, watching the breathing.

Follow-Up Activity:

Light your candle. Then, sit quietly, staring into the flame as you repeat your mantra. If you do not already have one, imagine a mantra (for instance, "Peace") and practice using it whenever you enter into meditations. Remember, your gratitude journal writing is a form of meditation that enables you to look within the depths of your soul. Master it. To follow the spiritual life as a caregiver, try to meditate at least once a day. It is best to meditate early in the morning when your world is calm and peaceful. Or perhaps in the late evening, or whatever time is more convenient to you. By giving importance to your meditation, your power of meditation will automatically increase.

WEDNESDAY, Week II

The fruit of silence is prayer. The fruit of prayer is peace.
—Mother Teresa

Yoga is a form of exercise that uses many meditation techniques, especially relaxation amid silence. It is practiced by many long-term family caregivers who have experienced the realization voiced above by Mother Teresa, and who are yoga students now engaged in helping others manage their excessive stress and promote relaxation.

Because we caregivers oftentimes live relatively isolated lives that keep us focused on the immediate needs of our loved ones, we can find yoga to be a haven. This is especially true when we are overwhelmed with demanding nursing responsibilities and in search for inner peace...a quietness of the soul.

Yoga is a method of silence that can be used widely by the family caregiver because it offers many meditation techniques. It is excellent for the mind, body and spirit. It helps with balance, strength, suppleness and coordination.

Some of the techniques we learn in yoga are posture, breathing control and self awareness that help us reach a state of super consciousness in which we feel as one in the heart of all creation.

In summary, yoga is a useful program of effective stress-reduction practices such as gentle stretching exercises, deep-breathing exercises, meditation and progressive deep relaxation for the mind, body and spirit.

Follow-Up Activity:

Do further research on yoga. Either find a yoga class in your community, visit the library and find a book about it, search for Internet sites on yoga or look for a yoga class on your television listing.

THURSDAY, Week II

Meditation is the pathway that leads to the inner self.

It is very important that we long-term family caregivers master the art of meditation because it takes us within ourselves, enabling us to know ourselves and use the knowledge for stress reduction and health promotion.

Meditation reveals to us that Spirit is the God part within us; the Mind is our capacity to use it, and Body is what results from that use.

Meditation tells us that the ultimate purpose of life always has been and must of necessity always be, to find God within ourselves in order to feel spiritually alive.

Meditation leads us in experiencing that we are one with all life.

Meditation awakens us to an awareness that our personal religion is the most important thing in our life.

Meditation guides us into achieving inner peace.

Follow-Up Activity:

Using your lighted candle, sit quietly and list as many gifts as possible that come from meditation. For example, meditation is good for stress reduction and health promotion. Record them in your gratitude journal. Continue to practice the gift of being silent.

FRIDAY, Week II

And ye shall know the truth, and the truth shall make you free. John 8:32

The gift of silence teaches us that one primary purpose of meditation is to rid the mind of limiting ideas, and free it for new concepts of truths that help us to know ourselves. Knowing oneself is a must for all caregivers.

Meditation is necessary in developing our recognition of the Inner Presence that gives light to our existence. We become fully aware that there is more to our existence than getting and having. We are here to spread love. Caregiving is the perfect opportunity to spread love.

Basically, meditation is the process of being still and freeing our minds for new insights that help unlock our inherited divinity. It enables us to see and feel the basic truth that we are one with the elements of the earth, and that it is up to us to live fully and abundantly. Meditation can also help us to know how we are to achieve all this.

When we meditate, we feel that God, the Infinite Intelligence and energy, is pouring into us, filling us with love's energy. The world spins on the energy of love.

In the silence of meditation we open up our consciousness to the flow of abundant life.

In the silence, we hear the whispered words: "I have come that they might have life, and that they might have it more abundantly."

In the silence, we become aware of our emotions and health, laughter and medicine, mind and body because they all come to focus, informing us that every education about life experiences is an inward journey.

Follow-Up Activity:

Note any changes in perception since you began this journey of using your spiritual keys to unlock your inner world. Write down ways in which meditation can help you know yourself and why you feel that this knowledge is of primary importance, especially as a caregiver.

SATURDAY, Week II

Blessed is the man that walketh not in the council of the ungodly, nor standeth in the way of sinners, nor sitteth in the seat of the scornful. But his delight is in the law of the Lord; and in his law doth he meditate day and night.
— Psalm 1: 1-2

Because caregiving is an experience that tests every fiber of the soul, the caregiver needs to follow a path of spiritual elevation which can better be accomplished through meditation...mind/body medicine.

One of the basic procedures for effective meditation might include:

(1) Relaxation - Let the body, mind and spirit become completely still.

(2) Expectation - Realize that something wonderful is going to happen.

(3) Recognition - Close your eyes, but focus them on a spot at the center of your forehead. Envision a soft light bulb pressed against your forehead. Imagine that it is the image of the song, "Lead, Kindly Light, Amid the Encircling Gloom." Let this kind and soft light suffuse itself through your entire being, warming and cleansing you. You feel inner peace. Feel the silence. Enjoy the light. Visualize and identify yourself with the light, then blend into it, unifying with your higher self as the silence whispers "Be still and know that I am God." Feel the love and joy that God is in everything and everything is in God. Enjoy your soul's journey as it follows the light, winging your flight over mountains and through valleys, over oceans and through green pastures where love is the only answer to any question you may have. In other words, you lose yourself in the meditation.

Follow-Up Activity:

Continue to practice the meditation technique daily, and as you grow stronger and stronger in its path you will feel the greatest joy and inner peace imaginable. Meditate by candlelight as often as possible.

WEEK THREE

Viewing Family Caregiving as a Spiritual Mission

The spirit of man is the candle of the LORD.
Proverbs 20:27a

When we view life's experiences in the context of a loving plan that has been devised for our growth, this understanding constitutes the greatest spiritual support imaginable. —A. Johnson

SUNDAY, Week III

Prelude

Athirst and with humility, the traveler prayerfully asked, "Oh, Divine Master, how can my disabled brother teach me that caring for him is a spiritual mission when it entails so many stressful responsibilities that test every fiber of my soul?"

With kindness and compassion, the Master replied , "My child, caring for your disabled brother is a mission that will teach you how to cultivate "God's Virtues" —the fruit of the spirit. But, first, you must be quiet and in your silence, listen attentively."

Love is the Greatest Creation of Life

But the fruit of the Spirit is love, joy, peace, longsuffering, gentleness, goodness, faith, meekness, temperance: against such there is no law. —Galatians 5:22-23

The *fruit* of the Fruit of the Spirit begins with love.

Basically, there are nine powerful graces given, and of these nine, the prophet Paul puts love at the top of the list. Love is the first in that beautiful cluster of delicious fruit;

and *gratitude* is the energy surrounding it.

Caregiving experiences teach us that all the other eight ingredients can be defined in terms of *love.* Joy is love that makes us feel happy and grateful; peace is love that gives us contentment; longsuffering is love that gives us courage to triumph over adversity; gentleness is love that instills in us the spirit of kindness and compassion; goodness is love in action; faith is love that helps us to believe, perceive and achieve our goals; meekness is love that gives us humility; temperance is love that teaches us self control. So, all the nine graces have their roots in love.

Love is the master key, the great motive, the essence of life.

When love is always the only answer, what then is the question?

There is no question because we can see from experiences that caregiving is a spiritual journey in which the Master is ordering our steps in the "Word" of love.

Follow-Up Activity:

When you adhere to these principles of love, you will find that they can combat caregiver-burnout. Try to start your day of family caregiving on a set of godly character development values that include the fruit of the spirit. Feel the joy that is building within you. Feel the spiritual growth as it fills your heart with gratitude. Record your thoughts, feelings and actions in your gratitude journal. Try doing this one day at a time until it eventually becomes a spiritual habit. Light a candle for each of the nine virtues. Sit quietly and stare into their flames, meditating for at least ten minutes.

MONDAY, Week III

Kindness is the True Universal Religion

Howbeit when he, "the Spirit of truth, is come," he will guide you into all truth. —John 16:13

In caregiving, we learn that the Creator (Love) speaks to us through human experiences, showing and telling us by our own everyday examples that kindness is the true universal religion. We can transform the world through kindness, one deed at a time. Kindness is spiritual.

In my life as a long-term caregiver, I find this to be one of the most powerful truths that has kept me focused on being Christlike in my daily attitude. Kindness is holistic medicine for the mind, body and soul.

If we love life, we know that greater than life is our personal relationship with God, who commands us to love one another; to be kind to one another. We are to always treat others with kindness, just as we wish to be treated, especially as caregivers. All religions throughout the world teach this basic, universal truth...Christianity, Judaism, Islam, Buddhism, Hinduism, Sikhism, and even the world's newest major religion, the Baha'i' faith that believes in the unity of all religions, the oneness of God and that ushers in an age of peace for all humankind.

Family caregiving teaches us that everyone wishes to be treated with *kindness*, love and compassion. When we love the Creator and obey His Commandment to love one another, we experience the highest joy we could ever achieve. We have awakened and are overwhelmed with the feeling of inner joy that floods our souls.

Family caregiving is a human experience of life. Therefore, when we view caregiving in the context of the

Creator's plan, we can begin to see it as a spiritual mission that enables us to cultivate kindness, love and compassion for others.

When we are able to see caregiving as a spiritual mission spreading kindness, we will feel the spirit of love within that will enable us to perform our responsibilities beautifully. We will experience the joy and calmness of inner peace as we continuously embrace the fruits of the spirit and meditate often each day on how to speak, think and act kindly.

Follow-Up Activity:

Light your candle. Then begin writing your thoughts and feelings about viewing caregiving as a spiritual mission of kindness. Be sure and write from the depths of your heart because you are in conversation with your inner self that speaks only truth. If the very idea seems outrageous, just work with it and allow it to lead you. Notice what thoughts, feelings and acts of kindness emerge that can transform your world. You may use the following example:

As a family caregiver, I can show my love through kind deeds by:

1. Cultivating a love that overflows in the spirit of kindness.
2. Performing works of mercy and compassion.
3. Using kindness in correcting others.
4. Recognizing the healing power of kindness.

TUESDAY, Week III

"I sought my God and He withdrew from me; I sought my soul, and it eluded me; I sought my brother, in him I found all three." —Anonymous

If we can view caregiving as a spiritual mission of kindness, it becomes a learning institution in which we continue to grow stronger and stronger each day. Caregiving, simply, is a growth experience that gives our lives meaning and purpose. Caregiving is a private school named Opportunity that teaches us by example how to serve one another with kindness, humility, joy and gratitude.

Because family caregiving can and does test the very fibers of our souls, we gain strength from the myriad of experiences when we let ourselves learn, with humility, what our disabled love one's illness is trying to teach us.

In the midst of crushing and relentless suffering, we will receive spiritual elevation. We will learn how to cope, how to keep moving on, and how to use our faith while living with the harshest of realities...the disability of our loved one.

On the journey, we must remember that caregiving and anger can sometimes seem to be inseparable. Sometimes anger flashes without warning.

Anger is an emotion that does not obey the rules of logic. This is where our quiet meditations come in with the spiritual strength we need to abate caregiver burnout. In the spirit of kindness, we must try to see ourselves in our loved ones. When we do this, we cannot harm him or her. Actually, we are all one in the spirit of love and kindness.

Follow-Up Activity:

Light your candle of kindness. Using your first name, keep

repeating silently this sentence that comes from your higher self: "Caregiver______, see yourself in others; who then can you harm?"

Write down some of the things your loved one does that angers you. See the anger as excessive stress that can be detrimental to your health or your loved one's health. While meditating, ask your higher self how can you best handle the anger and establish or restore your inner peace.

WEDNESDAY, Week III

They that wait upon the Lord shall renew their strength; they shall mount up with wings as eagles, they shall run, and not be weary; they shall walk, and not faint.
—Isaiah 40:31

We caregivers want to do more than merely cope with the overwhelming experiences of ever-mounting stress. We want to seek new and effective ways of taking control of our lives, preventing diseases that stem from stress, and enhancing our spiritual, mental and physical health to avoid heart attacks.

Those who are spiritually successful seem comfortable in almost any situation because they see caregiving as a spiritual mission. Their lives are full and yet unhurried. They look confident and relaxed, even when they are engaged in custodial care for their loved one or making crucial decisions. Being physically fit and seldom weary and tired, they project a sense of quiet strength.

According to social psychologist David Myers, an expert on happiness, spiritual people are happier. They are aware that their attitudes can belong to two families: namely, the faith family and the fear family. Basically, spiritual people choose to align their attitudes with the faith family.

Anger is a destructive emotional attitude that belongs to the fear family. We can get rid of a destructive emotional attitude by consciously developing the opposite, constructive feeling. So, we change families. We change anger for calm, fear for faith, confusion for composure, hate for love, dread for anticipation, depression for elation and resentment for forgiveness.

We can never be relaxed or balanced as long as we hang on to negative, destructive feelings. Such feelings can trigger "caregiver-burnout", heart attacks and a host of other debilitating ailments.

When we consider that we all are spiritual beings having human experiences, not merely human beings having spiritual experiences, we can readily see that all of us belong to the faith family that embraces the fruits of the spirit....God's treasury of virtues.

Follow-Up Activity:

Look at your life and view some experiences in light of the faith family. Light a candle. Afterwards, list some experiences in light of the fear family. Write them in your gratitude journal. Thank yourself for this awakening, then invite the faith family to live in your caregiving world forever so that you can always experience inner peace.

THURSDAY, Week III

A wise man will hear, and will increase learning; and a man of understanding shall attain unto wise counsels.
—Proverbs 1:5

Caregivers become angry even under the best circumstances. Expect it of yourself and don't be surprised by it. Don't try to deny its presence. How you face and manage your anger determines whether you will make it productive or destructive.

The following are some of the typical sources of anger for caregivers:

1. Your pertinent plans, goals, or expectations are delayed or deleted because you had to devote all your space to caregiving.
2. The duration, expense or difficulty of family caregiving.
3. The long-standing, unresolved conflicts of the disabled person.
4. Disagreements with the ill person or family members regarding treatment.
5. Your sense of helplessness in alleviating the loved one's suffering.
6. Financial problems that continue to mount due to medical expenses.

Mismanaged anger harms your well being and your relationship with your loved one. It creates and intensifies the myriad of problems you face when you as a caregiver lose control. That is why it is wise to meditate so that you can see the problems in the quiet place of your higher self. Remember, *a wise man/woman will hear and increase learning.*

Follow-Up Activity:

Analyze your present undesirable feelings and decide what their opposite, constructive attitudes are. Use every means at your disposal to develop good feelings, instead.

FRIDAY, Week III

Wisdom is the principal thing; therefore get wisdom: and in all thy getting get understanding. —Proverbs 4:7

Constructive management of anger can help you resolve conflicts and make peace with, forgive, achieve closeness with, or show compassion toward your loved one.

The following are a few ways in which you can accomplish this:

1. When you want to use your anger for problem solving, calm yourself by taking a few deep breaths and collecting your thoughts. Ask your higher self: "What do I wish to accomplish in this situation, or at this moment, that I'm not accomplishing?"

2. When you are angry, admit it to your higher self, not your loved one or others. Find a quiet moment, then meditate. A wise answer to the questions you may be asking, such as, "How can I find the spiritual message?" or, "How can I find help?" will be revealed to you in your silence.

3. With your loved one, explore solutions to the problems that cause anger if he/she is able to think clearly with you. Try to have this conversation when you are calm, not agitated.

4. Develop a variety of safety valves through which you can discharge your excessive anger. Always meditate, remembering your spirit. Also engage in exercises such as walking or running.

This is an excellent time to realize the wisdom and importance of feeling grateful, and how the feeling can create in your heart the spirit of joy and humility. *Feel* the joy of *feeling* compassionate. Remember, Eternal God is compassionate, and He breathes His energy of love and compassion within you. Oftentimes some religious ministers seem to paint God as a brutal protector. But you have the choice of seeing your God as a personal God of wisdom, love and compassion. *Feel* His love within you as it calms your angry attitude and you enter into His peace. Meditate always.

Follow-Up Activity:

Consult your higher self for wisdom and write down ways in which you can cultivate the spirit of more love and compassion for your loved one.

SATURDAY, Week III

Wisdom's ways are the ways of pleasantness, and her paths are peace. — Proverbs 3:17

Attitude is everything.

Gratitude journal writing and family caregiving experiences prove this universal truth in our everyday thoughts, feelings and actions.

When anger dominates our mind, the best part of the human brain, which judges situations, fails in its function. We may use hateful words unintentionally. Harsh words pour out automatically due to fear and lack of control when we cannot manage a stressful situation. Once the angry attitude subsides, we feel ashamed of ourselves.

We feel ashamed of ourselves because anger (feeling hateful) is not our true nature. Wisdom tells us that love is our true nature. Our eternal, peaceful home.

A negative attitude is negative energy. It is filled with fear and is contagious.

A positive attitude is positive energy. It is filled with love and is contagious.

You can exchange a negative attitude for a positive attitude through deep breathing. Taking in love and breathing out hate/anger.

You can do this by visualizing or training the mind through focusing on the object of meditation, keeping in view the fruit of the spirit...Love.

Remember, we are spiritual beings having human experiences. We are not human beings having spiritual experiences.

Our human experiences teach us by example that caregiving is a spiritual mission that enhances spiritual growth when we treat others as we would have them treat us. We all want to be treated with kindness. Remember the adage: "See yourself in others, who then can you harm?"

Remember, there is a difference between care taking and care giving. The following insight will help you realize the difference:

• **Care Taking:** *Problem Solving*: As the care partner talks, you are figuring out the problem and coming up with a solution. • **Care Giving:** *Listening*: Hears the problem, empathizes and makes observations.

• **Care Taking:** *Judging*: Beginning a sentence with "you should" or "why don't you." • **Care Giving:** *Sharing*: Says, "I'm here for you. Is there something I can do for you?" Shares something of self.

• **Care Taking:** *Peace Maker*: Trying to appease emotions, especially anger, by fixing the problem or figuring out how to avoid it, with the care partner or other team members. • **Care Giving:** *Truth-teller*: Is honest about difficult emotions, both the care partner's and her/his own.

• **Care Taking:** *Fixer*: Doing tasks that the care partner may not really want or need done. • **Care Giving:** *Giving*: Does something for the joy of doing it to foster companionship or friendship.

• **Care Taking:** *Helper*: Seeing yourself as stronger, more able, better equipped to help. • **Care Giving:** *Equal*: Sees the care partner as another person; just like me.

• **Care Taking:** *Superman/Superwoman*: Can do many things, and in the beginning tries to "do it all," but gets burned out and discouraged in the long haul. • **Care Giving:** *Healer*: Knows her own wounds and weaknesses; takes care of himself and uses these limitations to create a bond between himself and others.

Follow-Up Activities:

Light your candle. Write down ways in which caregiving has given you the opportunity to cultivate kindness through love and compassion for your loved one. You may never have thought about your service in this way before. Trust that you will see these fruits of the spirit, however small they may seem to you. Can you feel grateful for these experiences? Why should you see caregiving as a spiritual mission that promotes spiritual growth? Write down your true feelings. Spiritual growth is painful, but the rewards are absolutely beautiful!

WEEK FOUR
Cultivating the Spirit of Gratitude

The most perfect prayer is a sincere "Thank You" raised to heaven in the spirit of love. — Father Damian

SUNDAY, Week IV
Prelude

And then the enlightened traveler humbly asked in a prayer of meditation, "O Master of love and kindness, how can my disabled brother teach me the power of being grateful?"

"My child," the kind Master tenderly whispered, "he will teach you through your everyday experiences as a caregiver that gratitude is the foundation of human happiness, inner peace and prosperity. But you must listen, my child, in quietness and in solitude, for clear instructions."

The Gift of Gratitude

Give thanks always unto God and the Father in the name of our Lord Jesus Christ. — Ephesians 5:20

Gratitude journal writing teaches us through our own personal caregiving experiences that gratitude is the foundation of joy and inner peace. It is the pathway to God.

It is the key that unlocks the doors to a spiritually, morally and financially abundant life.

Caregiving is a spiritual mission that teaches us the power of gratitude. We are at our finest when we can give thanks in the midst of our trials and tribulations, our sadness, sufferings and our adversities.

Even though suffering is a choice, the wisdom of love is born in suffering.

Father Damian, an outstanding young priest at the Veterans

Administration Medical Center in Miami, Florida, told us family caregivers one day that the most perfect prayer is a sincere "Thank You" raised to heaven in the spirit of love and humility. He called gratitude "the mark of a truly noble soul."

God answers the soul's attitude, not the words. We should pray only for values, not for things; for spiritual growth, not for gratification.

We must remember that prayer is designed to expand insight...to expand our consciousness and enhance our spiritual perception. With this insight, we should cultivate an attitude of gratitude because it is the spiritual source of all happiness.

Follow-Up Activity:

Light your candle. Then, in your gratitude journal, list at least ten things for which you are grateful. Let some of them include your caregiving experiences. Meditate on them and say "THANK YOU" to your Creator (Love) for the experiences sent into your world of caregiving to help promote spiritual growth and to guide you in entering into His peace.

MONDAY, Week IV

In everything give thanks; for this is the will of God in Christ Jesus concerning you. Quench not the spirit.
—Thessalonians 5:18

Gratitude journaling and family caregiving experiences teach us that being thankful helps us to return to our natural state of joyfulness and abundance.

It enables us to see that adversity is a loving plan, and that we should be thankful for the experiences that propel our spiritual growth.

Yes, our disabled loved ones as well as the sick and

helpless people throughout the world are here to teach us to love, serve and feel universal compassion. Family caregiving brings the world to our doorsteps. We awaken and embrace it with His love that is planted within us all.

As caregivers, let us be grateful that the Master has entrusted the world of our disabled loved ones in our care, for it is in helping others that we are filled with the joy of inner peace on our spiritual journey.

Being our brother's keeper, life teaches us by human experiences that we are interrelated, interconnected and interdependent because we live in His world of commodities and services. Life's wisdom teaches us that God is in everything and that everything is in God...including commodities and services. When we help one another, it gives us the height of joy we all seek. It has been said that the way we treat others is the way we treat our personal God.

With an attitude of gratitude, let us not deny ourselves thc joy of loving, respecting and appreciating others in obedience to His command, so that we can experience inner peace and abundant life.

Follow-Up Activities:

Light your candle and in the silence, stare into its flame and feel the spirit of gratitude. Meditate. Think of at least ten (10) examples that convey how you, along with other human beings in this world, are interrelated, interconnected and interdependent. (Examples: equipment and services. Also...parents who bring us into the world and care for us; religious ministers who give us spiritual guidance; doctors and nurses who attend our illnesses; political leaders who are our local, state and national caregivers). Later, record them in your gratitude journal and, as often as possible, continue to add more to the list.

TUESDAY, Week IV

And he said unto me, "My grace is sufficient for thee, for my strength is made perfect in weakness."
— 2 Corinthians- 12:9

When my husband and I wrote our first book, *Mysterious Stranger Aboard, chronicling* our 40-year battle with multiple sclerosis, which is sometimes called MS, we profiled the human experiences of our triumphs over adversity. The book described our frustrations, depressions, exhaustion, anxiety, guilt, anger; and our loss of privacy, future plans, economic security, health, family and work.

It also showed how we began journeying through the pain by writing gratitude journals, a wise suggestion made by talk show hostess Oprah Winfrey. As a result, our spirit of gratitude made us think less but realize more. The writing increased our knowledge and expanded our insight. We were mysteriously and joyfully awakened to transcendent wisdom and universal compassion. En route, we have been abundantly blessed...spiritually and financially. In gratitude, we are now wonderfully engaged in works of philanthropy. Caregiving awarded us with its gift certificate of passion, perseverance and possibility...all enclosed in the envelope of love with the stamp of Eternal God.

On the journey, we have not only embraced the scripture quoted above with gratitude, which is worth repeating: "My grace is sufficient for thee, for my strength is made perfect in weakness," but my husband and I also blended our spirits with the rest of that passage scripture: "Most gladly therefore, will I rather glory in my infirmities, that the power of Christ may rest upon me." —2 Corinthians 12:9.

We are grateful for the voyage, the victor and the victory.

We are grateful for Oprah Winfrey who was, and still is, instrumental in encouraging positive change in our lives.

Follow-Up Activity:

Light your candle of gratitude. Meditate in your quiet space about experiences that have changed your life since you became a family caregiver. Afterwards, write some of them in your gratitude journal. Feel free to add more to the list as often as possible.

WEDNESDAY, Week IV

God saves the unfortunate through their affliction and instructs them through distress. —Job 36:13

Like the biblical character Job, we must be thankful for the gift of spiritual growth that leads us forward when adversity, chronic illness, clinical depression, physical pain, sorrow, distress, failure and temporary defeat overtake us.

With wisdom, understanding and gratitude we, like Job, can see that God saves us through our affliction and instructs us through distress.

Through prayer, meditation and gratitude journal writing we can see our own spiritual growth take wings. In essence, life is about growth. The first miracle of life is the law of growth (popularly known as evolution) through eternal change.

G .... God (Love) first. • Give gratitude to the Creator for life and His creation.

R .... Religion. • Be grateful for your religion. Kindness is the true religion.

O .... Obey. • In gratitude, obey God's will to love one another.

W ... Witness. • In gratitude, be a witness for love and service to others.

T ..... Thankful. • Be thankful in all things. Make thanksliving your attitude.

H .... Holy Spirit. • Be thankful that we have hope in the Blessed Trinity... The Father, Son and Holy Spirit. A mystery.

Let us be thankful that we are evolving. And let us be thankful for the presence of the Eternal Father in our lives as we view our human experiences in the context of His loving plan. And because we know that spiritual growth is born in suffering, let us in love, humility and gratitude whisper, *Thy will be done.*

Follow-Up Activity:

Light your gratitude candle, and in your quiet space stare into its flame and meditate on experiences in your life in which you were saved through affliction and instructed through distress. Believe me, they exist. Afterwards, record at least five (5) of them in your gratitude journal and express your feelings of joy and thankfulness. In your daily world, practice saying "Thank You" as often as possible, and note how you feel and what wonderful things happen as a result.

THURSDAY, Week IV

Gratitude journal writing is the key to locked up blessings and an abundant, joyful life.
— "O" Magazine

When we learn to tap the miraculous power that lies within our own grateful personality, everything we desire will be within our reach.

Human experiences have taught us that success belongs to people who cultivate a life of *thanksliving*. The November 2000 issue of *"O"* magazine has shown us outstanding individuals who have cultivated a life of thanksliving. To these individuals, spiritual and economic abundance is a daily miracle...a way of life.

Throughout the ages, life has shown us that success belongs to those lucky people who are blessed with successful personalities of gratitude. Wise people in every successful profession have learned to achieve their goals, to overcome adversities and obstacles to their success, to live the abundant life of love and service through the miraculous power that comes from an attitude of gratitude.

Oprah Winfrey has stated that she has spent a lifetime being grateful, and that is why she was so happy to present the contents of November's magazine to her readers as we celebrated the month of Thanksgiving. She wrote that being thankful is an art to be cultivated and practiced from moment to moment; and that appreciating what we have changes our perception of what we think we need.

Follow-Up Activity:

Go into your quiet space, light your candle and think of experiences in which your being grateful has brought you abundant blessings and success. Write them in your gratitude journal.

FRIDAY, Week IV

Not that I speak in respect of want: for I have learned, in whatsoever state I am, therewith to be content.
— Philippians 4:11

Mother Teresa once said, "She gives most who gives with joy."

Gratitude for small things makes every day a sacred gift with joy.

When we look to others for joy and fulfillment, we will never truly be filled. If the experience of happiness depends on financial wealth, we will never be happy with ourselves because we will always want more.

When we are content with what we have, we can be thankful and feel fulfilled. We can rejoice in the way things are.

When we realize that there is nothing lacking, and that everything is just as the Creator planned, the whole world belongs to us.

We can create our own happiness by creating our own perceptions, projecting an attitude of gratitude. We also can find happiness in the sheer joy of being alive and in the sweet fellowship of others regardless of faith, race or nationality.

Feelings of gratitude actually promote good health by releasing positive chemical compounds called endorphins throughout the body. When we cultivate an attitude of gratitude, we are growing our souls to heal our wounds that stem from being ungrateful.

Gratitude gives birth to positive feelings: love,

compassion, joy and hope.

When we focus on the many things for which we are thankful, any negative feelings of fear, bitterness, jealousy, selfishness and ego-tripping vanish.

Happiness is less a matter of getting what we want than wanting what we actually need. What we actually need is an attitude of gratitude. A spirit of gratitude makes us stop whining and start shining.

Follow-Up Activity:

Review Thursday's journaling. Then staring into the flame of your gratitude candle, meditate by thinking of five or more reasons why feeling grateful makes you happy. Record them in your gratitude journal.

SATURDAY, Week IV

Be careful of nothing; but in every thing by prayer and supplication with thanksgiving let your request be made unto God.
—Philippians 4:6

Love cannot be far behind a heart that is thankful and a mind that is grateful. There is not a more pleasing exercise of the mind than gratitude. Life is a miracle. A miracle is a universal blessing from God; and that miracle should always inspire gratitude. Let us be thankful for the miracle of life. When we cultivate the spirit of gratitude, we experience the simple joy of living from a grateful heart. Attitudes of gratitude enable us to give and receive joy every day of our life, no matter what is going on.

Below are some of the gifts of gratitude we have identified in our caregiving experiences that promoted our inner peace.

Let us try to embrace them with a thankful attitude and **feel the love** within our hearts.

Gratitude is the joy of *feeling* the presence of Eternal God in our lives.

Gratitude is the *feeling* of love, kindness and humility in action.

Gratitude is the mother of joy and inner peace.

Gratitude promotes good mental and physical health.

Gratitude promotes our spiritual, social and economic growth.

Gratitude is a positive attitude filled with positive energy.

Gratitude makes us feel young at heart and joins us to all life.

Gratitude eradicates worry, stress, depression, caregiver burnout.

Gratitude draws people to us and connects us to spirit.

Gratitude gives us a spirit of love, service and compassion.

Gratitude enables us to truly see caregiving as a spiritual mission.

An attitude of gratitude has enabled us to see and appreciate life as a precious gift. Can you see this gratitude attitude as providing blessings for you? In gratitude for this gift, we can gladly make our lives a blessing to others. In so doing, we make our lives a blessing to ourselves and to our Creator.

Follow-Up Activity:

Enter into your quiet space and light your candle. Stare softly into the flame and begin meditating on the kindnesses that stem from being grateful. In what ways can you make your life a blessing of kindness and compassion to others, including your disabled loved one? Think humbly, then in your gratitude journal, make your requests to God.

Journal writing is really a powerful type of meditation and carries many of the same benefits. A journal makes us aware of how active our minds are while we are paying no attention to our thoughts, as when we shower or eat. A gratitude journal can make us become conscious of all these ideas and learn from them. Just writing the words is not enough, however. Really concentrate on the words as you write. Watch how you feel about what you are writing.

WEEK FIVE

Identifying the States of "Caregiver-Burnout"

It is more than right that we thank God unceasingly for you...because your faith grows apace and your mutual love increases. —2 Thessalonians 1:3

SUNDAY, Week V

Prelude

In the spirit of gratitude, the humble traveler silently prayed, "Kind Master and keeper of my soul, please tell me how can caring for my disabled brother teach me the wisdom of long-term caregiving so that I will not be a victim of caregiver-burnout?"

The Master kindly replied, "My child, He will teach you through family caregiving experiences how to recognize the stages of caregiver-burnout. You may use the wisdom and continue the spiritual journey of kindness, love and service as I have commanded. But first, you must be quiet, meditate and attentively listen."

Touching Lives, Lifting Spirits

While sharing my gratitude journal, *Caring for the Caregiver,* with Mrs. McQuire, a high school teacher, and her students who were filming the event, she handed me the following article entitled "Caregiver" taken from the March 27, 2001, issue of *Daily Word.* She commented that we caregivers share a common bond that helps us to avoid "caregiver burnout."

> *With a heart of love, I reach out tenderly and compassionately to others.*
>
> *When people need special care because they cannot care for themselves, I may find myself asking, "God, what can I do that would be of help?"*

God's answer resonates within the silence of my soul: "Dear one, there is a divine purpose that is already unfolding through you. You are answering the call to be a caregiver. Let your love and compassion guide you and help. As a caregiver, you are willing and able to share the limitless love and compassion that are within you."

It is true. God has given me a heart of love, love that has the power to reach out tenderly and compassionately to touch others. The words I speak encourage and motivate others to heal. My actions comfort and console, for I am a caregiver.

"Love one another. Just as I have loved you, you also should love one another." —John 13:34.

Yes, family caregivers share a common bond... touching lives, lifting spirits. In order to find excitement everyday in our lives, we befriend and share our experiences with others who have similar responsibilities. Friends are important to caregivers because they are a source of refuge and strength to those who are trying to avoid caregiver-burnout.

Follow-Up Activity:

In what way does this article fit into your life as a caregiver? Write your responses in your gratitude journal.

MONDAY, Week V

When wisdom entereth into thine heart, and knowledge is pleasant unto the soul; discretion shall preserve thee, understanding shall keep thee. —Proverbs 2:10-11

The following coping strategies are excerpted from my gratitude journal, *Caring for the Caregiver:*

• Choose to take charge of your life, and do not let your loved one's illness or disability always take center stage. Protect your well-being and your selfhood.

• Remember to be good to yourself. Love, honor and value yourself. You are doing a very hard job and you deserve some quality time just for you.

• Watch out for signs of depression, and don't delay in getting professional help when you need it. Be aware of the emotional concerns of you and your loved one.

• When people offer to help, accept the offer and suggest specific things they can do. Promote participation in family relationships by designing a care plan.

• Educate yourself about your loved one's condition. Information is empowering.

• There is a difference between caring and doing. Be open to technologies and ideas that promote your loved one's independence and protect your well-being.

• Trust your instincts. Most of the time they'll lead you in the right direction.

• Stand up for your rights as a caregiver and a citizen. Seek moral and spiritual support from other caregivers. There is great strength in knowing that you are not alone. Balance caregiving and your selfhood.

• Grieve for your losses, and then allow yourself to dream new dreams. Always remember the age-old adage: "In reality, nobody belongs to us, except in memory."

Follow-Up Activity:

Can you think of coping strategies that have worked for you as a caregiver? In your gratitude journal, record at least five of them and write "Thank You" because now, you are beautifully evolving.

TUESDAY, Week V

Frustrations and sadness are the most frequently felt caregiver emotions. —National Family Caregivers Association

Experiences have shown us that negative feelings of frustrations and sadness can trigger excessive stress for the individual. Because these negative feelings are most frequently present in the life of a family caregiver, they can cause caregiver burnout, making it impossible for the caregiver to spread kindness.

"Caregiver-burnout" is an illness we want to avoid. Although we have been told that some stress is unavoidable, we need to know as much as possible about the excessive stressors in our daily life.

Basically, we know that stress is not inherent in an event, but rather in how an individual *perceives* that event. Therefore, let us perceive our mission of caregiving in a manner that will help us overcome caregiver stressors that trigger caregiver burnout.

First, we need to be aware of danger signals.

Caregivers must learn about the stressors in their lives,

and practice the art of relaxation so that, in life's mission, they can spread the seeds of kindness.

It is imperative that caregivers know how to overcome special stressors, such as those created by caregiving as presented later in this section.

The caregiver must be knowledgeable about attacking the stressful behavior, the thoughts, attitudes and actions that occur as a result of caregiving.

The caregiver should plan her/his days carefully in order to encourage balance that will enhance good physical and mental health.

The caregiver should meet with support groups that consist of other caregivers and medical experts, and learn of information regarding caregiving in various settings (i.e., in home, in-patient, nursing home, long distance, hospice care, etc.).

The caregiver, in the spirit of kindness, should help his/ her loved one to feel very special. Caregivers may practice the habit of feeling grateful to the Creator for the opportunity to serve.

Follow-Up Activity:

If you have never attended one, make plans today to attend a support group. Whether you have or have not attended such a group, write your thoughts and feelings about attending a support group of family caregivers. Record them in your gratitude journal for further consideration.

WEDNESDAY, Week V

More people enter nursing homes because of caregiver burnout, rather than an exacerbation of their own physical condition. - National Family Caregivers Association

Caregiver-stressors that trigger caregiver burnout come in four stages. These stages, that seem to slowly emerge like a thief and destroy one's peaceful state of mind, may be identified as follows.

(1) The Beginning Stage of Caregiver-Stressors:
- (a) The continuous interruption of ideal plans.
- (b) A myriad of pressing obligations.
- (c) The need for urgent decisions.
- (d) The increase in stressful behavior, thoughts and attitudes.
- (e) The occurrence of disbelief and shock.
- (f) The family's need to adopt a new theme.
- (g) The anxiety of trying to put it all together.
- (h) The importance of communicating your needs and feelings.
- (i) The importance of evaluating the stressors in your new life as a caregiver.

(2) The Stage of Complications:
- (a) The inconveniences of human experiences.
- (b) The need to readjust your schedule.
- (c) The stress of continuously explaining to others.
- (d) The urgent struggle to recognize plans.
- (e) The constant hope that things will get better.

Follow-Up Activity:

Write down your thoughts and feelings regarding stages one and two. How many of these caregiver-stressors have you experienced and how have you handled them? Light your candle and meditate on these experiences.

THURSDAY, Week V

The thief comes only to steal and slaughter and destroy,
I came that they might have life and have it to the full.
- John 10:10

(3) The Stage of Pressure:
- (a) The occurrence of family conflicts.
- (b) The lack of some form of resolution.
- (c) The flare-up of a mild form of depression.
- (d) The sign of physical stress.
- (e) Impatience over small stuff.
- (f) The lonely feelings of withdrawal and isolation.

(4) The Stage of Burnout:
- (a) The occurrence of physical illness.
- (b) The threat of family disruption.
- (c) The possibility of separation.
- (d) The reappearance of serious symptoms.
- (e) The feeling of severe depression and despair.
- (f) The anxiety of wanting to escape or run away.
- (g) The habit of drinking to escape the stress.
- (h) The occurrence of uncontrolled violence to end the stress.

Follow-Up Activity:

List some of the experiences stated in stages 3 and 4 that

you have encountered and/or are now encountering. Tell how you handled them. Write your responses in your gratitude journal. Light your candle and meditate deeply on them.

FRIDAY, Week V

And he said unto me, Son of man, stand upon thy feet, and I will speak unto thee. —Ezekiel 2: 1

Learning to be strong by standing upon your feet and speaking up is the lesson to be learned by caregivers who want to care for their mental, physical and economic health and peace of mind. Try to follow these guidelines to help promote a sense of well being and inner peace. Remember, attitude is everything.

(1) Practice the art of doing one thing at a time. It has been said that doing one thing, while thinking about ten other things that you should be doing, is extremely stressful. Make spending relaxing quality time with your loved one a priority.

(2) Set reasonable goals for yourself. Don't form the habit of making an impossible list and then feel stressed when you don't get it all done. Do some of it at another time. Move along with nature for, her pace is patience.

(3) Try to avoid feeling that everything is so very grave! This stressor is caused by the thought that whatever we are doing is very serious. Just remember that feeling this way doesn't make us more responsible, it just gives us more fuel for becoming a victim of caregiver burnout.

(4) Laugh and play more. Be optimistic. Think positive. Happy thoughts can alter attitudes and enable you to enjoy your world of *thanksliving* with your loved one.

(5) Spend and save money wisely. Remember, anybody can spend money but many do not know how to spend it

wisely. The ability to spend and save money wisely is a test of your economic wisdom. In regards to saving money, remember the adage: *It is better to have it and not need it than to need it and not have it.*

(6) Secure the professional services of a financial advisor.

Follow-Up Activity:

Light your candle and sit quietly, staring into its flame and meditating on additional ways in which you can care for yourself. Afterwards, get your gratitude journal and list activities that will bring laughter and that feel like fun. Can any of these activities be undertaken with your loved one participating? If not, make a list of fun things in which you feel he/she can participate even in the silence of the mind. For instance, using your imagination, you can envision your body swimming peacefully across the ocean and feeling as one in the heart of all creation. You can envision yourself being an eagle, flying far above the clouds, winging your flight over all the earth. You can envision your spirit traveling to other planets, enjoying the beauty and holiness of all creation. You can travel vicariously to all areas of the world, meeting people of all nationalities and feeling the joy of brotherly love and compassion. Imagination is Love's magic gift in action. It is God's perfect gift to us.

SATURDAY, Week V

Many times, caregivers put so much emphasis on their care recipient's health that they neglect their own.
—National Family Caregivers Association

Caregivers need to know that protecting their own health must be their highest priority. They are the pillars that support their families. When they become ill or disabled, everything falls apart. Caregivers need to stay healthy for themselves and their disabled loved ones. They cannot afford the luxury of getting sick, but it happens. "You may think one catastrophe per family is enough, but illness is no respecter of the law of averages," writes NFCA in its *Take Care* newsletter.

NFCA notes that the prime areas you need to be concerned about are your own health, your support team, and your insurance coverage. These three areas should be immediately evaluated.

(1) *Protect Your Own Health.* • Get a checkup. Make an appointment with your doctor for a complete physical. If you are ignoring symptoms, now is the time to get them checked. • Take care of yourself. Even if you get a clean bill of health from your doctor, don't be complacent. Are you overweight? Are you exercising regularly?

(2) *Line Up Your Emergency Support Team.* • Who will be the surrogate caregiver? • Develop an emergency support system; divide the responsibilities in sections. • Put emergency system agreements of the surrogate caregiver's responsibilities on paper.

(3) *Evaluate Your Insurance Coverage.* • Health Insurance. • Catastrophic Coverage. • Medicare. • Disability Insurance. • Long Term Care Insurance.

Performing these priority responsibilities will combat excessive stress, abate "caregiver-burnout" and promote inner peace for both the caregiver and her/his loved one.

Follow-Up Activity:

If you haven't already done so, prioritize your own health by taking care of yourself: body, mind, and spirit. Visit your doctors as often as necessary and try to follow their orders. Develop an emergency support system of family and friends who can help with the responsibilities of caregiving. Review your insurance policies immediately. Write in your gratitude journal how you plan to take care of yourself in your everyday experiences that will help you avoid "caregiver burnout."

Make sure that all of your entries include a variety of "thank you" phrases that project your gratitude for the gift of life and all creation.

WEEK SIX
The Spiritual Gifts of Family Caregiving

Though I speak with the tongues of men and of angels and have not love, I am become as sounding brass or a tinkling cymbal. — 1 Corinthians 13:1

SUNDAY, Week VI
Prelude

Finally, and with a heart of humility and gratitude, the traveler silently prayed, "O, kind and loving Master, my disabled brother has taught me through caregiving experiences that all things in creation are holy, even the ugly, violent and incomprehensible. Please tell me now how can he teach me that family caregiving is a spiritual gift from You?"

Smiling compassionately, the Master softly whispered, "He can teach you the principles of faith, hope and love, my child. And you will learn through caregiving human experiences that the greatest of these three principles is love. Be grateful, my child, to your disabled brother for teaching you the pathway home. Now, through deeds of kindness, you can share his teachings with others and enter into my rest."

Love is our Spiritual Home

The spiritual gift of family caregiving is the experiences of practicing the elements of *kindness by caring for our brother*. Love is our spiritual home because it is God's kindness in action toward our fellow man.

Kindness is the voice of the soul. The soul speaks; we listen in the spirit of love and kindness...lovingkindness.

There is nothing in this world more beautiful than loving God (Love) and obeying His will to love one another. Over and over again, life experiences teach us by example that kindness is the truest religion because it has all the ingredients of love...our spiritual home. When we understand that love is our spiritual home, and that the only way we can arrive "home" is through the deeds of kindness we show toward our brother.

Family caregiving is a ministry that enables us to experience this state of kindness. It enables us to climb to the highest levels of unconditional love through kindness to one another. No man can stand so tall as when he stoops to help the disabled.

With this insight, we realize that family caregiving is a magnifying mirror that reflects our truest selves and that enables us to return to love.

The many experiences of family caregiving clearly teach us that love is, indeed, our spiritual home.

Follow-Up Activity:

Light your candle and enter into your quiet world. Meditate for at least five minutes about your family caregiving mission and your spiritual home of love. In what ways can you make your caregiving a ministry? Some of the ways you might consider may include: (1) sharing your knowledge of "the wisdom and joy of expressing gratitude," (2) sharing with others the joy of living in kindness, love and service to humanity, and (3) engaging in volunteer services at hospitals, nursing homes and other service facilities.

List your ideas in your gratitude journal and mediate on them, letting your higher self give you more spiritual insight into your thoughts and feelings.

MONDAY, Week VI

And though I have the gift of prophecy, and understand all mysteries, and all knowledge; and though I have all faith, so that I could remove mountains, and have not love, I am nothing. —1 Corinthians 13:2

Gratitude journaling reveals to us: (1) we do not see things as they are; we see things as we are, and (2) attitude is indeed everything. We are our attitudes.

Family caregiving gives us the opportunity to develop an attitude that projects the ideal qualities of freedom, responsibility, courage, love and inner integrity.

One might say that these are qualities that are never perfectly realized by anyone, but they are the psychological goals which give meaning to our movement toward the integration of social justice, universal peace and brotherly love.

Family caregiving is a rich source from which to draw a wealth of knowledge that can be used to realize these qualities.

Jesus of Nazareth said, "Follow me." He taught us by human examples how to unlock our inherited divinity with the power of kindness and unconditional love. We must learn to meditate at all times on His teachings of love and service. In meditation, we blend our spirit with His spirit and feel the joy of being one with Him and with our personal God.

This gift of caregiving's transcendent wisdom and universal compassion can be shared with all society, showing others that we meet God in our love for one another.

When Socrates was describing the ideal way of life and the ideal society, a student said, "Socrates, I do not believe that there is such a City of God anywhere on earth." Socrates answered, "Whether such a city exists in heaven or ever will exist on earth, the wise man will live after the manner of that city, having nothing to do with any other, and in so looking upon it, will set his own house in order."

"Follow me," Jesus said to my husband, our MS and me when the three of us were searching for God to help us courageously live with the debilitating illness that seemed bent on destroying us...body, mind and soul. So now we joyfully follow Jesus because He is the answer. The overwhelming thirst for God is one of the spiritual gifts of family caregiving. Finding Him in our brother is the way that leads directly to Him.

I shall never forget the weekday morning when I was driving home from mass with radio station WMCU (Miami Christian University) turned on and listening to Steve Brown and his "Key Life" commentary. Ironically, for two days I had been agonizingly disturbed over my awakened frustrations as to whether Jesus was "God" or "The Son of God." Suddenly, the voice on the radio said, "...and now many of you Christians are yet confused and wondering was Jesus of Nazareth 'God' or was he the 'Son of God'. Well, let me tell you my friends that according to Scripture, Jesus is the Son of God. **Jesus is God Incarnate!"**

Actually, I was so shocked that my soul's attitude was suddenly and beautifully answered, that I almost wrecked the car. Then I wondered was my life an illusion. I hurried home, grabbed the dictionary from the office library shelf and defined the word *incarnate.*

Incarnate *- embodied in flesh; invested with a bodily, esp. a human, form... (2) personified or typified as a quality or idea.*

Well that was all I needed to know because in my world,

Jesus is *God and God Incarnate*. The Word made flesh. More important to me was dedicating my life to follow His teachings because He is the answer. He is love. Inasmuch as love is the only answer, what then is the question?

Neal Maxwell, an Apostle of the Church of Jesus Christ of Latter Day Saints, tells us that when Jesus said in the New Testament, "I have other sheep not of this fold," He was referencing the people here in America. Elder Maxwell further stated that there will be a great winding up when Jesus comes again not in the meekness of the manger, but in majesty and power. "And it will come in a time of great tribulation, including in Jerusalem. And so all of His purposes will be achieved."

Let us quote from the Lord's prayer to Our Father:

Thy kingdom come, thy will be done
on earth as it is in heaven.

Follow-Up Activity:

Light your candle and stare into its flame, meditating. In the quietness of your mind, think of ways in which the experience of family caregiving is teaching you by human examples the wisdom and joy of love and kindness. Afterwards, list them in your gratitude journal. Do you see a difference in your thoughts and feelings concerning this experience, from those you held when you first began reading this book?

TUESDAY, Week VI

And though I bestow all my goods to feed the poor, and though I give my body to be burned, and have not charity, it profiteth me nothing. —1 Corinthians 13:3

The National Family Caregivers Association wisely urges caregivers to protect their own health and to give it their highest priority. They warn that caregivers need to stay healthy for themselves and for their loved ones.

Why is it so important for caregivers to consider their own health their highest priority? Is this self love?

Father Damian has explained the why of this counseling more emphatically.

He stated that if anyone will not learn from the lessons and teachings of Christianity to love *himself* in the right way, then neither can he love his neighbor in the right way. To love one's self in the right way and to love one's neighbor are absolutely analogous concepts...they are one and the same. Hence, the law is: " You should love yourself as you love your neighbor when you love him as you love yourself."

Consciousness of self is not introversion. Caregivers should not try to forget themselves by locking their feelings in an attitude of self-consciousness.

Self-consciousness is identified with morbid introspection, shyness and embarrassment. You do not wish to be labeled as such. It is important to be conscious of ourselves to the point of being self-confident. To be merely an observer of ourselves, to treat ourselves as objects, is to be a stranger to ourselves. Those who don't love themselves as they actually are rarely love life as it is, either.

Consciousness of self actually expands our control of our lives, and with that expanded power, we have the energy to let ourselves rise to our highest potential.

The greater self-consciousness one has, especially the caregiver, the more spontaneous and creative she/he can be at the same time, unlocking her/his inherited divinity.

Follow-Up Activity:

As a family caregiver, in what ways are you conscious of self? Your gratitude journal should, by this time, offer you a clear picture of your inner self. If so, what do you see? What would you like to see?

WEDNESDAY, Week VI

Love suffereth long, and is kind; love envieth not; love vaunteth not itself, is not puffed up, does not behave itself unseemly, seeketh not her own, is not easily provoked, thinketh no evil. — 1 Corinthians 13:4-5.

One of the spiritual gifts of caregiving is that it provides caregivers with an opportunity to *feel* the unconditional love within ourselves. Without feeling the spirit of love within ourselves, long term caregiving responsibilities can make our thoughts, feelings and actions ungodly. We are our religion; and the perils of long term caregiving puts it through a series of spiritual testing experiences.

Knowing and *feeling* are two different activities. Basically, we are thoughts and feelings. These two powerhouses are stored inside our actions.

Thoughts are wonderful; but feelings are the seat of the soul. When we feel the love within our selves, it is our soul in action. Love, not thought, is the greatest creation of life. Jesus of Nazareth taught us this truth by example. He was, and still is, the greatest teacher who ever lived. He taught us how to live even amid suffering.

"'Follow me,' Jesus Christ said," counseled Fathers Damian and Fernandez of the Veterans Administration Medical Center to us caregivers and our disabled, war veterans. We embraced their counseling because caregiving teaches us that the central purpose of Jesus' life was to destroy the life of loneliness and to establish here on earth the life of love. Caregiving provides an opportunity for the caregiver to follow the wisdom of love and humility taught by Jesus Christ, the incarnation of God.

Christianity is the religion founded upon the life and teachings of Jesus Christ. It has spread throughout the world, and is the prevailing religion in the Western Hemisphere. Christians make up the largest religious group in the world, numbering more than 860 million. Christianity has influenced government, thought and art for almost two thousand years. It is now influencing science, holistic healing and caregiving.

We *feel* the love and we ask the Creator to guide our steps in the Word that teaches the wisdom of love because it brings us joy. Caregiving teaches us that joy gains its glory out of sorrow, bitter sorrow and human loneliness. This is why caregiving experiences show us that the central purpose of Christ's life, indeed, was to destroy the life of loneliness and to establish here on earth the life of love. *His law is love and his gospel is peace.*

Follow-Up Activity:

In what additional ways do you view caregiving as a spiritual mission? Review your Sunday, Week VI activity and temper these ideas with your other lessons. Record your response in your gratitude journal.

THURSDAY, Week VI

Love rejoices not in iniquity, but rejoices in the truth; beareth all things, believeth all things, hopeth all things, endureth all things. —1 Corinthians, 13:7

Through deep meditation, we can find a center of strength within ourselves to face and conquer the insecurities of our world. We may even have to let go of our confused beliefs and ideas about life and other people that we have been taught in order to have a life. We should never deny ourselves the joy of loving others and the happiness of continued spiritual growth.

This is the wisdom of love that caregiving experiences teach. Mastering them, we experience inner peace. These experiences extend to us the opportunity to develop good social skills and interpersonal relationships, They provide us with the following commandments of human relations:

1. SPEAK TO PEOPLE. There is nothing more beautiful than a cheerful word or greeting that comes from the heart. It is love in action.

2. SMILE AT PEOPLE. It takes 72 muscles to frown; only 14 muscles to smile. "A frown has negative energy that is contagious to everything in its surroundings...even the window curtains, floor carpeting and dishes," my analyst once joked.

3. CALL PEOPLE BY NAME. The sweetest music to anyone's ears is the sound of his/her own name.

4. BE FRIENDLY AND HELPFUL. If you would have friends, be a friend. Friends are the masterpieces of nature.

5. BE CORDIAL. Speak and act in the spirit of love as if everything you do in the spirit of love is a genuine pleasure.

Follow-Up Activity:

Make a special effort to remember and practice these social skills with everyone you encounter today. The results will amaze you. Think of other social skills to add in your gratitude journal. Note the results of your social skills exercise.

FRIDAY, Week VI

Love never faileth: but whether there be prophecies, they shall fail; whether there be tongues, they shall cease; whether there be knowledge, it shall vanish away. ...For now we see through a glass darkly, but then face to face.
—1 Corinthians, 13:8, 12.

The gift of caregiving experiences exemplifies for us a known truth that when a person is locked up inside himself or herself, he or she makes a pretty small package. The following social commandments are continued from the previous page, and they highlight ways in which we can cultivate the joy of loving others.

6. BE GENUINELY INTERESTED IN PEOPLE. You can love almost anyone if you try. Love never faileth. Remember, everyone wants to be loved. This is a basic instinct that follows us from the cradle to the grave. Treat a person as though she/he is the most important person in his or her world. To you, you are the most important person

in your world. Every so often, surprise someone with a small gift or kind note of appreciation.

7. BE GENEROUS WITH PRAISE; CAUTIOUS WITH CRITICISM. Remember, everyone likes to feel that he/she is loved, appreciated, respected, important and special. Even you. Therefore, treat others as you would have them treat you.

8. BE CONSIDERATE OF THE FEELINGS OF OTHERS. There are usually three sides to a controversy: yours, the other fellow's, and the side of truth. Be a good listener, be understanding and forgiving.

9. BE ALERT TO GIVE SERVICE TO OTHERS. What counts most in life is what we do for others. When we help others, it gives us the feeling of heavenly joy we all seek.

10. ADD TO THIS A SENSE OF HUMOR, LOVE and an ATTITUDE OF GRATITUDE, and life will reward you abundantly. The universe always responds in kind to our attitudes. It is important that we always obey its law of cause and effect .

Laughter is Holistic Medicine

Laughter is oftentimes the best medicine. Sometimes we can even find laughter within our illnesses, disabilities and caregiving.

I am reminded of a serious conversation I once had with my husband about Jesus of Nazareth and His disciples, and how He ordered them to follow Him and He would make them fishers of men. In an even more serious tone, I told my husband that we must also be fishers of men.

My husband smiled and said in his stammering speech, "Yeah, Alice, we catch 'em and He'll clean 'em."

Laughing heartily, I replied, "You and your multiple sclerosis caught me and Jesus of Nazareth cleaned me, giving me a clean heart of love so that I could serve Him and be used by Him as your caregiver. And now we both are joyfully 'writing for Him' in gratitude for our spiritually, abundant life."

Folding in laughter, my husband said, "Now that MS and I caught you and Jesus cleaned you, the three of us (you, MS, and me) have gotta go fishing and catch some more 'burned-out' caregivers like you were and let the Master clean 'em, too, Alice."

Astounded that he responded so clearly, I continued with the humor. "Better still, I'd rather the Master clean MS, inasmuch as you've caught it and are still holding on to it while writing for Him."

He chuckled. Then nodding his head continuously, he said, "Alice, the Master said I didn't catch MS; it's a gene. He made my MS a lifeline to pull us aboard His peaceful shore, Alice. Didn't our gratitude journaling show us how MS went fishing and caught us and Jesus cleaned us with his wonderful power of love? You'd better always be grateful that 'He cleaned us,' Alice, and awakened us to 'feel the joy!'"

I shrieked, "Wow! John-n-n-n! When did you learn to talk in long, complete sentences like those? The only response I ever get from you is 'Oh, boy'."

"Oh, boy," he said and we both bellowed, catching our breaths only to continue the laughter. Again we saw that his illness, just as most other illnesses, is indeed a mysterious stranger aboard.

At that time, I was more shocked and excited about John's

returned voice than his wisdom. Why? Because even in his silence, his body language and two-word responses projected wisdom when we communicated.

This episode revealed to me that love and laughter, like gratitude journal writing, is mind/body medicine and good for the soul.

Follow-Up Activity:

Think of some humor you and your loved one have shared. Record some of the sweet memories in your gratitude journal.

SATURDAY, Week VI

And now abideth faith, hope, love, these thee;
but the greatest of these is love. —Corinthians 13: 13

In summary, scripture tells us that love is the greatest creation of life. It is greater than faith and hope. God is eternal love; God is eternal life. God is also energy. Energy cannot be created nor destroyed. We are the energy, breath and fragrance of God. *In Him we live, and move and have our being.—Acts 17: 28.*

God is a heart that contains all our hearts, a mind that contains all our minds, a voice enfolding all our voices, a silence deeper than all our silences, a love encircling all our love, a spirit enveloping all our spirits, a beauty more precious than all things beautiful.

Gratitude journal writing teaches us the gifts of family caregiving. It provides an opportunity for the spiritually orientated caregiver to walk humbly and without fear through the valley of the shadow of death and, though folded in tears, whisper silently from the depths of their heart: "Thy will be done."

Gratitude journaling teaches us that caregiving is a gift that shows us by example that everything starts with thought. Thoughts are responded to by feelings. Feelings build attitudes. The prevailing mental and emotional attitudes determine experience. Experiences form the pattern of our lives.

Caregiving is a gift that teaches us that love is the essence of life; life is a mystery to be lived; life is a series of problem-solving situations; life is a precious gift. We can avoid "caregiver-burnout" and find inner peace when we religiously:

(1) Practice the skills of stress management.
(2) Meditate daily and regularly.
(3) Continue to grow spiritually.
(4) Cultivate an attitude of gratitude.
(5) Establish good human relations.
(6) Feel God's presence within us and see caregiving as a gift.

Caregiving is a gift certificate inviting the caregiver into the kingdom of God by humbly and joyfully living the mystery and solving the series of problems life will present in the spirit of His love. It is a gift that gives us knowledge to teach on the platform of society. We gather caregiving experiences and present them to the world as sermons learned as we engage in the joy of *writing for Him.*

Caregiving is a gift that opens doors of opportunities for us to learn through experience that kindness is, indeed, the truest religion. It unites all religions. The spirit of kindness orders our steps in "The Word" of love as we enter into the kingdom of heaven. Here we see the face of God by touching lives and lifting spirits.

Follow-Up Activity:

In your program of abating "caregiver-burnout" and finding inner peace, you can reflect on the six tips given above in summary of the six-week activity. Light your candle and write down some of the things you learned by looking at your thoughts , feelings and emotions in retrospect. Be especially aware of how your thoughts, beliefs and feelings create emotions. Examine the positive emotions. Try to incorporate them in your everyday activities and record your progress. Although it is presented here as a six-week program, it is a lifetime commitment if you want to avoid excessive stress and experience the joy and contentment of inner peace and prosperity. Congratulations on your spiritual journey!

Epilogue

And the now awakened traveler took up her heavy cross and humbly followed the teachings of her disabled brother, seeing in her brother the Holy Spirit of the Master that dwells in all creation. In the quietness of her own soul, the traveler had found the commanding Master and had awakened Him. On the journey, the traveler learned that stress-control is Self-Control. Caregiving wisdom had taught her that Self-Control is Strength; Gratitude is Humility; Love is Mastery; Calmness is Power...altogether these lessons formed a combination lock code that opened the doors to love, abundant life and inner peace.

Overwhelmed with feelings of joy, the traveler folded in prayer as she entered into the Master's rest with praise, humility and gratitude, knowing that all creation is holy, even the illness of her disabled brother who taught her the wisdom of love.

We accept good things from God; and should we not accept evil? Job 2:10b

Thus, gratitude journal "Writing for Him" through family caregiving experiences can teach us all that kindness is, indeed, the true universal religion. The spiritual keys for avoiding caregiver-burnout and promoting inner peace are clearly bestowed when we cultivate the joy of Writing for Him.

Spiritual Key # 2

Gratitude: The Basis of Human Happiness

Enter into His gates with thanksgiving, and into His courts with praise, be thankful unto Him and bless His name.
Psalms 100: 4

FOREWORD

To become Christlike is the only thing in the whole world worth caring for; the thing before which every ambition of man is folly, and all lower achievement vain.
— Anonymous

Prelude

The traveler gently asked, "Kind Master, how can I become more Christlike in my world of family caregiving when I am always being confronted with adversities that disrupt my state of equilibrium?"

The Master smiled. "My child, listen quietly to your world of family caregiving and hear the echoes of each new day as your brother shows you the face of Christ. When you hear the melodious sonnet, light your candle and meditate on the harmony, then share its light with others."

About the Chapter

As a family caregiver, gratitude journal writing has taught me that there is nothing more beautiful than loving Eternal God and joyfully obeying His will to love one another. In doing so, we become Christlike.

Gratitude journaling is the miracle key to the myriad of locked-up blessings that can teach us caregivers the age-old truth: "kindness is the true universal religion."

Through human experiences reflected by gratitude journaling, wisdom has shown me that Eternal God answers our soul's *attitude* of humility, not our uttered, spiritless words.

For this reason we should pray for His help in cultivating an attitude of gratitude and kindness because prayer is designed to expand insight, to awaken us and to make us more realizing. An attitude of thankfulness and kindness gives life its true meaning.

When John was admitted to The Veterans Administration Medical Center Nursing Home because of severe multiple sclerosis, I was swept into feelings of chronic depression that overwhelmed me.

In spite of my many prayers and various other efforts to be Christlike and to combat the sadness, I tended to feel a tremendous loneliness and loss. I felt that only my being in the company of my husband could overcome these feelings. I did not understand at that time that the worst loneliness is not to be comfortable with yourself. Well, my inner self eventually told me that I was not comfortable with myself and that I needed to communicate in solitude with my higher self to overcome the sadness. In my cry for help, I communicated with my higher self through gratitude journal writing and, as usual, with my husband.

Mysteriously, the experiences of being near my husband and gratitude journal writing did eradicate my state of loneliness. How? Because John implied that oftentimes depression is a spiritual gift and suggested that I, quietly and humbly, listen to the inner message and pray for a spirit of gratitude. He told me that gratitude journal writing would put me in direct contact with the God within.

And it did. The experiences of multiple sclerosis showed us that gratitude is the mother of human happiness. "Gratitude gives birth to happiness just as a mother gives birth to her child and nourishes it," my husband had counseled years ago in the early stages of his illness. "Gratitude is one of the most happy feelings you will ever experience."

Gratitude is an Attitude of Choice

My husband also told me that gratitude is an attitude.

Prayer combined with gratitude journal writing, I learned from experience, is designed to, indeed, make us humans less thinking but more awakened. Prayer is designed to expand our insight into the past, present and future. Years of caregiving experiences taught me to pray for spiritual and moral values, not for things. The experiences of caregiving taught me to pray for spiritual growth, not for gratification.

I learned also that pain is inevitable; suffering is optional. Through gratitude journaling, life taught me by human experiences the age-old truth that "wisdom is born in suffering." When we read about the lives of outstanding men like Mohandas K. Gandhi and Martin Luther King, we see this basic truth. They were Christlike.

"Let gratitude become your way of life," my husband had softly whispered into my ocean of loneliness. Scripture tells us that Christ was forever giving thanks to God the Father.

Embracing my husband's school of thought, I began putting his wisdom to a test every time life's dark shadows imprisoned my world. While silently meditating, I could always hear a soft, compassionate inner voice whisper with the wisdom of love, "Be thankful always."

And now, when I feel depressed, I always listen to the quiet voice of the Creator within. While listening, I feel the message as I venture into life's series of problem solving situations that flood my world. Awakening to the spiritual message, expressing gratitude for the spiritual growth it entails as I adhere to it, I feel the love and the joy of experiencing life with passion and with happiness born of gratitude journaling.

On the journey of caregiving, wisdom from gratitude journal writing has revealed to us that when we meditate daily on our human experiences, we find that gratitude is Christlike. It is a beautiful and *mysterious stranger aboard* where *love paints beauty in the soul* with *symbols of love* amid *the calm and the strife* that create our world of family caregiving. Miraculously, in order to l*et your attitude be gratitude*, you must see and appreciate these symbols of love because, along with bringing happiness, they will show you by experiences that *love finds expression through kindness and concern.* By *caring for the caregiver,* the recipient of the care and our fellow man, we are being Christlike...spreading love and kindness. Thus, caregiving experiences and gratitude journal writing together show us that *we create our own happiness*, and that happiness is the goal of life. Family caregiving is a spiritual mission that teaches us by example the abundant joy and blessings bestowed on anyone who chooses to be grateful.

PART 1
God Answers the Soul's Attitude

But when thou prayeth, enter into thy closet., and when thou hast shut thy door, pray to thy Father which is in secret; and thy Father which seeth in secret shall reward thee openly. — Matthew 6:6

Prelude

The awakened traveler, desperately searching for more lighted candles from her disabled brother, realizes that on life's journey we are always arriving, yet we never arrive. Praying softly, she asked, "Kind Master, I have been faithfully following the teachings of my disabled brother and have experienced joy. But oftentimes, I feel very unhappy and I don't know why. Will he teach me how to always *feel* the happiness within?"

With a spirit of compassion, the kind Master replied, "My child, caring for your brother will teach you that *gratitude* is the basis of happiness. But you must first enter into your quiet space, light your candle, meditate and listen pensively to the messages his caregiving has taught you, over the years, about gratitude through your journal writing. Then, share its message with the world."

1. The Gifts of Gratitude Journal Writing

Gratitude is the mother of joy. Joy is prayer.
Joy is a net of love by which you can catch souls.
—Mother Teresa

Family caregiving experiences have taught me that gratitude journal writing is a silent prayer that mirrors the soul's thankfulness. It is a gift that blesses us with the opportunity to enter into the closets of our minds and talk with our higher selves from the depths of the heart, the seat of the soul. It unlocks the doors to abundant life...spiritually, physically and financially.

Because gratitude journaling reveals to us that the mind is a closet of thoughts and feelings, and that attitude is everything, the journaling becomes a lighted candle that sends its beams into the far corners of our closets, illuminating the attitudes that accompany our thoughts, feelings and actions.

The more I record life's experiences in my gratitude journal series, the more I realize the impact of attitude on human life.

Wisdom gained from gratitude journal writing has revealed to me that attitude is more important than knowing basic facts.

Gratitude journaling teaches us that *attitude* is:

- More important than the past, present or future
- More important than education
- More important than money
- More important than circumstances
- More important than failures
- More important than success
- More important than what people think, say or do
- More important than appearance, giftedness or skills.

Gratitude journaling teaches us that attitude can make or break a home, a church, a business or a life. Attitude is *your* spirit.

A negative attitude, if carried to the extremes, can result in a life of emptiness that is incapable of spiritual growth; it is a life of loneliness, disconnectedness, selfishness, greed, clinical depression, egomania, hatefulness, abnormal fear and suspicion, excessive stress, and can be fatal to one's health and life as well as the heath and life of others.

We are unable to change our past, nor can we change the basic fact that other human beings will act a certain way. It is impossible to change the inevitable. The only thing we can change is *our* attitude.

Gratitude journal writing is a miracle gift that can help us change our attitude to gratitude. The remarkable thing is, when gratitude journaling, we have a choice every day regarding the attitude we will embrace for that day. As a family caregiver, I am convinced that life is one percent of what happens to me as an individual and ninety-nine percent of how I react to it. This basic fact also applies to all of us. We are in charge of our attitudes because attitudes are shaped from within.

Therefore, it would benefit us profoundly to cultivate the habit of letting our attitude be gratitude, because gratitude is the basis for human happiness and the gateway to answered prayers.

Gratitude journal writing opens its doors of wisdom and teaches us from our own everyday experiences that gratitude is the single most important disposition to be cultivated in our life and world today. Through silent prayers, we can turn our thoughts into feelings of gratitude and experience the peace, joy and abundance an attitude of gratitude brings.

This is the miracle gift of gratitude journal writing that stems from the soul's attitude of thankfulness.

2. *Prayer and the Soul's Attitude*

We pray to our Father, the Creator of the soul. And in praying, our attitude speaks, revealing our thoughts and feelings. Thus, we are made aware that attitude is, indeed, everything.

When we pray, do we feel the love and gratitude that flow from our souls?

If our attitudes fail to project feelings of love and kindness within, and we are plagued with feelings of disillusion and ingratitude, we then need to pray for a spirit of gratitude. This action can best be accomplished through gratitude journal writing.

One of the *miracle* gifts of gratitude journal writing is that it teaches us by examples that a spirit of gratitude makes us happy.

We all want to be happy. We all want our prayers to be heard. Gratitude journaling speaks into the silence of our hearts, awakening us to our innermost thoughts and feelings, and thus bringing us in direct contact with our higher selves.

As a family caregiver who enjoys viewing The Oprah Winfrey Show because it offers spiritual support, I followed the suggestion she first made to us listeners years ago to keep a gratitude journal. In my experiences, I realized that gratitude journal writing is the epitome of silent prayers that come from the depths of the soul.

Gratitude journal writing that stems from family caregiving teaches us not to pray for things, but to pray for values such as kindness.

Gratitude journal writing teaches us not to pray for gratification, but for growth.

Gratitude journal writing is designed to make the caregiver less thinking but more realizing. Like prayer, gratitude journaling is not designed to increase knowledge but to expand insight.

Gratitude journal writing utterly changed my world of family caregiving. My essential attitude transformed from ingratitude to gratitude, enabling me to stop whining and start shining.

When we see caregiving as a spiritual mission that extends to us the opportunity to cultivate the fruits of the spirit, and when we record our thoughts and feelings in a gratitude journal, we are forever in communion with the soul.

3. Your Feelings of Doubt Prove Your Sincerity

While gratitude journal writing, you might question your own belief in God. Perhaps you have always doubted that there is a God. When you speak this truth to your higher self, you are being sincere. You are speaking from the heart. Don't be afraid of your doubtful attitude because gratitude journal writing will help you realize that doubt proves that you are sincere.

The opposite of doubt is faith. Even people who are considered to be atheist believe in something. Gratitude journaling helps you to find the thing that you love and begin building from that point. This feeling of love is the way to the divine. This feeling of love that you *feel* within you is God. Remember, God is love and his spirit dwells within you.

Keep writing in your gratitude journal about all the symbols of love that have come into your life: (i.e., food, shelter, clothing, people, etc.). Write about all the wonderful, positive people who have shown kindness and compassion toward you and who have made your journey easier. In gratitude journaling, try to accentuate the positive and eliminate the negative. *Your focus is to highlight the love that flows in your world and that you have been too blind with negative attitudes to see.* Gratitude journaling will help the acts of love to surface. When you begin sincerely counting your blessings and awakening to all the wonderful people who have shown you acts of kindness and love, you will be astounded and filled with gratitude.

Oftentimes without doubt, there can be no faith. Therefore, recognize and respect your doubts, examine them and your attitude, and ask the spirit of love to consume your thoughts, feelings and actions, and to help you to *feel* the love within. In so doing, you will find that love is your soul's true home.

Suddenly your heart will open and you will know that God is real. Without the mind, the heart cannot hear. First the mind must be open, then the heart. Without an open mind, the heart cannot hear. Gratitude journaling gives you an open mind, a direct path to the heart.

Let your spirit of gratitude take you home, to the seat of your heart where love is always the only answer to any question. We must learn to listen to life appreciatively. We must listen to the lives of other outstanding role models whose world of doubt have been miraculously changed to a world of faith because of unceasing prayers.

4. A Classic Example of Gratitude Journal Writing

Let me seek you, Lord, by praying to you and let me pray believing in you, since to us you have been preached.
—St. Augustine

If you have read *The Confessions of Saint Augustine*, the story of Augustine of Hippo (354-430) and his early life and conversion to Christianity (a classic example of gratitude journal writing), you will recall with love and compassion how the doubt he described was changed to unshrinkable faith with such fervor that he was made a saint after his death.

In his book, he spoke of his early life in which he desperately searched for truth and in which he doubted God's substance or what way led or led back to Him. He told how his mother, Monica, a devout Christian, fervently and humbly prayed for several years that he would stop doubting God's nature and be converted to the Christian faith. With an attitude of humility, gratitude, faith and unconditional love for God, she prayed non-stop a mother's prayer for the conversion of her son. Oftentimes, she prayed silently, knowing that prayer is the soul's sincere desire, unuttered but spoken in the silence of the heart.

In response, and in His own time, when Augustine was ripe, our compassionate and loving Eternal God answered the soul's attitude of Augustine's tearful mother. In quietness and in solitude, while Augustine was still silently meditating in search for truth, his heart suddenly opened and he knew that God is eternal life and his spirit dwells in the heart of all His creation! Augustine's heart exploded with joy because he had found the pearl of greatest price, he wrote. He was awakened and enlightened by the spirit of Divine Intelligence. On the wings of joy, he girded his flight into the spirit of Eternal Truth and Love.

In gratitude for this divine response to his mother's prayer, and for the unspeakable joy of being awakened to divine truth, Augustine gladly and humbly dedicated his life and talents to love and serve God. He learned to love God with so much passion that he became an outstanding Christian theologian. His brilliant mind produced many great writings in defense of the church. Some of his writings are still being used today. His book, *The City of God*, is a defense of Christianity and the Catholic Church. Augustine knew that his brilliant mind was a direct line of creation, from God through him to all mankind. With this wisdom, Augustine was humble before God, yet great in Him. We see this spirit of humility and greatness throughout all his works, especially in his classic autobiography, *The Confessions of Saint Augustine*.

In the introduction to *The Confessions*, writer Rex Warner tells us that we see the story of a man who journeyed from sin to sainthood, from heresy to the heights of theological insight, from the darkness of worldly ambition to the changeless light of grace.

St. Augustine, in his desire to listen to life appreciatively and with humility, ranks first among the early fathers of the church.

Because St. Augustine's overwhelming love for God has always impressed me to the point of folding in tears of joy and gratitude, I was astounded to learn that we both were born August 28. When I am writing in my gratitude journal, I often feel the presence of his humbling spirit of wisdom, love, gratitude and kindness.

In prayers or meditation, I thank Eternal God for role models like Jesus of Nazareth and St. Augustine who showed us how to listen to life appreciatively and with humility so that we, too, can follow the path that leads to His kingdom of love and inner peace.

5. *Listening to Life Appreciatively*

Giving thanks always for all things unto God and the Father in the name of our Lord Jesus Christ.
—Ephesians 5:20

Inasmuch as gratitude journaling mirrors the soul, I humbly thank the Creator for awakening me, through myriad overwhelming experiences of intensive family caregiving, that gratitude is the mother of human happiness and the key that unlocks the doors to abundant life.

From the depths of my heart, I am grateful for the Creator's quiet whisper of love on that painful day eighteen years ago when I, tearfully enraged and chronically depressed from caregiver-burnout, attempted to throw His Holy Bible into the wastebasket. Depression punctuated by frustrations, doubts and a painful search for truth led me to perceive the Holy Bible as merely an anthology of Jewish history. In my cry for help that day, God answered my soul's attitude by softly and tenderly whispering the words of His beloved son, Jesus of Nazareth, *"Follow me."*

In solitude, the words of Jesus move us, who thirst to follow his teachings and listen to life appreciatively, to awaken us to His message:

The thief comes only to steal and slaughter and destroy.
I came that they might have life and have it to the full.
— John 10:10

Chronic fear and doubt that stemmed from "caregiver-burnout" was the thief that came to steal, slaughter and destroy my faith in the Heavenly Father's eternal love, kindness and compassion. With humility, I am grateful to Him for revealing to my troubled mind, amid the trials and tribulations of family caregiving, and the kindness and concern of hospitals' and nursing homes' medical staff members, that an attitude of gratitude is the most direct line to Eternal God and our inner peace.

In my endeavor to listen to life appreciatively, and to write about the experiences in a gratitude journal, love has shown me that caregiving is a spiritual mission that teaches us the transcendent wisdom and joy of unconditional love and universal compassion, and that we are at our finest when we can give thanks in the midst of our trials.

Gratitude unlocks the fullness of life and turns our assets into enough, and more. In our answered prayers that stem from the soul's attitude of gratitude, we find that gratitude turns denial into acceptance, chaos into order, confusion and frustrations into clarity. The spirit of gratitude makes sense of our past, brings peace and joy for today, and creates a vision of continued spiritual growth and beauty for tomorrow. Prayers of gratitude bring miracles to lay before the gates of heaven.

When we listen to life appreciatively, we are awakened to the wisdom of Jesus of Nazareth when he said, "The kingdom of heaven is within you."

When we listen to life appreciatively like St. Augustine and others who show their love for God and neighbor through acts of kindness, we find that heaven is a song of gratitude, love and praise.

When we listen to life appreciatively, we can make our professions ministries that spread love and kindness to all humanity.

6. Make Your Job a Ministry

What is heaven but a song of gratitude and love and praise by everything created to the Source of its creation?
— A Course in Miracles

When my psychologist informed me that I have creative writing skills, I immediately began developing them, and writing became an obsession. I began writing for God in search of myself and, astoundingly, I found God within me and my neighbor. When I was awakened to this joy, I fell in love with the spiritual journey because it is the pathway to contentment, happiness and fulfillment. My choice was to make inspirational writing a ministry. Family caregiving with its experiences of pain and suffering, joy and sorrows, fear, love and tremendous spiritual growth provided the foundation.

When I discovered that God dwells within me, my neighbor and all creation, I could not help but keep singing:

What a wonderful change in my life has been wrought since Jesus came into my heart; I have light in my soul for which long I have sought....Floods of joy, O my soul, like the sea billows roar.

Other songs overwhelm me such with such lines as: *He *touched me, and O, the joy that floods my soul; *Light of my soul, my joy, my crown; *This little light of mine, I'm gonna let it shine; *Those who see light can walk in the dark; *We are the light of the world, may our light shine before all that they may see the good that we do and give glory to God.*

If you recognized your oneness with God, you would know His power is yours. In gratitude for this power, you would humbly thank Him and ask Him to help you use this power to spread kindness and love.

We all have been given a special gift to be used for utilizing this power. We will know that our profession is a gift, if we have a passion for it. If we do not have a passion for it, even after praying for spiritual insight, then the job in which we are engaged may not be our mission... our spiritual gift.

With this perception, we should pray again from the heart, asking the Creator to help us awaken to our mission... our passion in which we can shine His light of love and kindness into the heart of all creation.

In gratitude for our job, we can make it a ministry by spreading love and kindness in the workplace. Responsibility makes us perform our duties; love makes us perform them beautifully.

Normally, people do not associate their jobs with love and kindness because jobs have come to be regarded as simply tools for making money. If you have this attitude, then you need to begin writing gratitude journals and get to the root of why you are here. Gratitude journaling will reveal to you that you are in this world to heal and be healed. Spiritually orientated people are not in the business of working only to make money; they are in the business to help bring love and kindness into the world. Making money is secondary and is to be used wisely to finance life and help bring love and kindness into the world.

A job is a gift. The reason God gave us a passion for the gift is because He wants us to perform that specific task for His kingdom of love in which we humans are interrelated, interconnected and interdependent. We humans are co-creators of the universe, and we must "be about our Father's business," to paraphrase Jesus.

Our Creator gave us the joy of engaging in our gift with a passion that no other job could possibly give. Our rightful job was singled out especially for us and it came with a passion especially made for us, and with a mission assignment especially given to us. Thus, we have our spiritual mission with its ingredients of abundant love, passion, joy, economic security, peace and contentment. In performing our rightful job—which is our gift, we are given a great opportunity to cultivate the fruits of the spirit, namely: love, joy, peace, longsuffering, gentleness, goodness, faith, meekness and temperance.

In gratitude for His gift, we should perform our jobs in the spirit of love, kindness and humility. Gratitude journaling reveals this awakening.

Subsequently, gratitude journal writing gives us a passion for humbly speaking from the depths of our hearts. Writing in our journals is the spirit of silent prayer and meditation. It is spiritual psychotherapy. When we develop a passion for praying humbly, we will experience that God does answer our soul's attitude.

Have you ever asked yourself why do you have a passion for your work? It is because God wants you to love and enjoy your gift. He wants you to be happy. The gift is His love to you. When you use it to spread love and kindness toward others, your using it in this manner is your gift to Him. Remember, when we pursue our spiritual mission with a passion, we find that genius is ninety-nine percent hard work with a passion and one percent skill.

The Creator's Commandments that we love God and our neighbor as we do ourselves is His ultimate gift to us. When we obey these two commandments, we experience the greatest joy imaginable. Loving God and obeying His commandments give us the joy and inner peace for which we all thirst.

When we make our jobs our ministries, we will learn the secret power of having an attitude of gratitude. Our prayers will be answered when our attitudes meet the petition of our spirits and not just the petition of our mere minds.

When we make our jobs our ministries, our ministries become a direct line of creation, from God through us to all humanity. Thus, the world will beat a pathway to our door. People will seek us out. We then experience abundant life.

7. Gratitude Journal Writing is Unending Spiritual Growth

The wisdom derived from gratitude journaling teaches us that genuine prayer adds to our spiritual growth, enables us to cultivate an attitude of gratitude, guides us in the path of humility, gives us that joy that comes from community with divinity, and awakens us to see genuine prayer as a spiritual-growth stimulus. Genuine prayer is a spontaneous outburst of God-consciousness in which we are fully aware of the presence of the Spirit of God to whom we fervently pray: "Thy will be done."

One of the major gifts of gratitude journal writing is it teaches us that genuine prayer is not a way of escape from human suffering but rather a stimulus to spiritual growth, in the very face of suffering. Because the caregiving experience teaches us to pray only for values, not things; for spiritual growth, not for rewards, it certainly develops the power of genuine prayer to all who utilize prayer.

In addition, caregiving experiences teach us that the word value of prayer is mostly autosuggestive in private settings and sociosuggestive in group settings. For this reason we can understand why Eternal God responds to the soul's attitude, not the spiritless words. Praying is a personal experience designed to adjust the personality to the will of God.

Fortunately, gratitude journaling reveals to us that the universe is unfolding as it should. When we view life's experiences in the context of a loving plan, and we let our hearts humbly whisper, "Thy will be done," prayer is the calm expression of gratitude and praise. Therefore, ninety-eight percent of our prayers should be prayers of gratitude and praise. Two percent can be used for making our requests known to God.

With this awakening, we can substantiate why gratitude is a direct line (e-mail) to our Creator.

8. *Humility of the Soul*

"Humility is the soil of the garden of the soul,
the good ground on which the divine Sower
goes forth to sow His seeds.
— Fr. Cajetan Mary da Bergamo

Gratitude journaling teaches us, especially the caregiver, that humility is the soul's strength and the ultimate secret of the spiritual life of being grateful. It is the alphabet out of which every virtue is formed and built up. It is a jewel because when we embody it from the soul, we neither underestimate nor overestimate our life. It is the expansion of our consciousness.

Humility, the God-life within us, is our feeling of consecrated oneness with humanity. "Be humble in God, yet great in Him."

Our ego talks; our humility acts. The ego, which is the little "i", is very limited and is constantly seeking something for itself. The large "I," the Larger Self, is not seeking anything, for it embodies everything within itself and belongs to the Infinite, the Eternal and the Immortal. It cares for the full perfection of God's entire creation.

When we serve soulfully, there can be no pride because we do not feel superior; instead, we feel humble because we are serving the Supreme in others. True service is rendered with humility and it comes only with true and constant aspiration and gratitude.

Gratitude journal writing awakens us to the wisdom that our talents are a direct line of creation, from God through us to our neighbors. It teaches us that a proud attitude is destructive, and that we can cultivate humility of the soul by expanding our knowledge of:

- The virtue of humility by subjecting ourselves to God and eradicating self pride
- Humility towards our Creator by expressing the soul's gratitude for His gifts
- Humility towards neighbor through acts of kindness, appreciation and respect
- Humility toward ourselves by giving God the glory and honor for everything.

PART 2

Gratitude: A Mysterious Stranger Aboard

Be careful for nothing; but in everything by prayer and supplication with thanksgiving let your request be known unto God. —Philippians 4:6

Prelude

Feeling humbled by what her chronically ill loved one had taught her, the awakening traveler felt a deeper thirst to understand the mystery of being grateful. "Kind Master, in my busy world of unending responsibilities of caring for my brother, how can he teach me the mystery of gratitude?"

"You must continue to meditate and quietly listen to your busy world of experiences, my dear child," replied the kind Master. "Through caregiving and gratitude journal writing, your eyes will open and you will see the mystery and abundant blessings of being thankful. When you see them clearly, you must share your light with the world."

1. The Mystery of Being Grateful

Delight thyself also in the Lord; and He shall give thee the desires of thine heart. —Psalm 37:4

When love is always the only answer, what then is the question? Gratitude is known to be one of love's great mysteries. Flowing from the fountain of love, gratitude is indeed the most humbling and beautiful "mysterious stranger aboard" our lives that makes it possible for us to feel the spirit of kindness within. With its majestic power, gratitude lights candles of love in the dark rooms of our hearts.

When our spirits live in our lighted rooms of thankfulness, we will be abundantly rewarded by the amazing, universal law of cause/effect. We will be given the desires of our heart.

Gratitude is a magic *feeling* of love that brings pleasant memories into our consciousness. Gratitude has the magic of making us feel grateful for the gift of *feeling* thankful no matter what happens in our lives. If we want to be happy, we must be grateful.

Caregivers know that it is not easy to be grateful all the time, but it is the times when we do not feel grateful that we are in desperate need of what being thankful can offer us. The magic of being grateful paints beauty and abundance in the soul.

Gratitude is a cleaning solution for the soul, healing our attitudes from the inside out. When we express gratitude for an act of kindness, the positive effects expand within our thoughts and feelings.

Our feeling of gratitude is a mysterious stranger with blessings locked up inside the garden of abundance, both spiritually and financially. Caregiving experiences have the keys for unlocking the gates of the garden and entering into the mystery of its magic through acts of kindness.

Gratitude journaling reveals to us that when we humans, misunderstandingly, deny ourselves the joy of *feeling* grateful and *feeling* unconditional love for one another because of fear, selfishness and ingratitude, we are denying ourselves the joy of feeling love and gratitude for ourselves.

Gratitude is a mysterious stranger that helps us to *feel* unconditional love for the Creator and all His creation, especially for one another and for ourselves.

Gratitude is a mysterious stranger that opens our hearts, enabling us to wisely respect organized religions and conclude that whether or not a person is a religious believer does not matter much. Far more important is that his/her attitude is one of love and kindness.

Gratitude is a mysterious stranger aboard that reveals to us the wisdom that kindness is the true religion, and that we should be thankful for all acts of kindness because of its universal healing power. It can heal the disease of destruction and war in the world.

Gratitude journaling provides for us the opportunity of awakening to the world of kindness that surrounds our everyday experiences. While it is true that we allow our busy agendas to block our visions for seeing the acts of kindness and love that surround us, the universe continues to bless us with its many gifts because we are loved, unconditionally, by our Creator.

I appreciate the kindness of Fr. Edwin Hayes of Christ the King Catholic Church in Miami, Florida, for wisely informing us during one of his sermons that: "God doesn't love us unconditionally because we are good, God loves us unconditionally because God is good."

Therefore, we must learn, by being grateful, the wisdom of forgiveness and compassion just as God forgives and shows compassion, because forgiveness is a form of gratitude. When we forgive and have compassion for others, we show them the mercy that we have often received and for which we are thankful.

Life is mysterious. And like life, gratitude is the mysterious stranger aboard that teaches us, through gratitude journal writing, that if we consider the world's major religions from the widest perspective, we find that they are all directed toward the spirit of gratitude. They all believe in the oneness of God who has given us the Commandment to love one another in the spirit of His kindness. They all believe in loving and giving thanks to the glory of God for the gift of life and for His universe. Such major religions as Christianity, Judaism, Buddhism, Hinduism, Islam, Sikhism, Zoroastrianism, the

Baha'i faith and others are all dedicated toward helping human beings follow God's law of love and kindness.

The magic of gratitude journal writing shows us the mystery and joy of being grateful. Through gratitude journaling, the experiences of caregiving teach by examples that ingratitude is the basis of human unhappiness.

2. Listening To The Inner Voice via Gratitude Journal Writing

"In quietness and in solitude, we hear His voice."

As I was writing in my gratitude journal this morning, October 9, 2000, after listening to the news that portrayed a world of crime, I realized how much we blundering society of humans owe our Creator an attitude of gratitude for life itself. But according to the news media, ninety percent of Americans are far too busy to pray or give thanks. This, I feel sure, is the reason for our accelerated crime rate. Mothers killing their children, children killing parents, children killing children, parents killing parents, simply a startling number of people killing people is getting to be more and more shocking and disturbing.

The spiritual message from these preposterous murders tells us that our ingratitude for the precious gift of life is the basis of human unhappiness. There is a strong need for us to cultivate the habit of saying prayers of thanksgiving. We are here to spread love, not hate; to be kind, not evil.

Gratitude journal writing is a tool that can help add to our prayers of thanksgiving and kind acts of *thanksliving*. It allows us to listen to the silent voice of kindness within us.

This valuable lesson is one I learned in my many visits to the hospitals and nursing homes where I saw love and service in action...people helping people, especially the helpless, just as the Creator commanded us. People "doing the will of God." *Be ye kind to one another.*

The inner voice of gratitude journaling whispers into our silence and says in the spirit of kindness and love: " Be still and know that I am God."

In listening, we hear a spiritual solution to our social and economic problems. In listening, we become more receptive or understanding as our insight expands. In listening, we feel the peace that passes all understanding.

Gratitude journaling is a gift that unfolds for us the mystery of being grateful. And as we become more realizing and our insight expands, we discover that God is in everything and that everything is in God. Remember, gratitude journaling is spiritual psychotherapy for the soul. Our souls need healing, and we are here to help each other heal.

When we listen to the silent voice within, we can feel the love, and thank God for the gift of life by making a firm decision to live it productively.

We can begin living life productively by keeping a gratitude journal to record our productivity as we live in the space of thankfulness.

In the silence of our minds, we can thank God for our talents and our abilities by accepting them as spiritual missions to be invested for the betterment of humankind.

We can express our attitudes of gratitude to Eternal God for all the kind things that courageous men and women have done to help us by doing kind things to help others.

In our gratitude journals, we can thank Eternal God for family caregiving experiences by accepting them as a challenge for achieving a higher level of opportunities, understanding, compassion and gratitude.

As we listen to the inner voice while writing in our

gratitude journals, we can thank God for kindness by helping to make the world kinder.

We can express our gratitude to the Creator for the creative ideas He has given us that enrich our lives by contributing these creative ideas to humanity.

In the quietness of the soul we can listen to the inner voice and express our attitude of gratitude that writing in a gratitude journal is a rewarding activity. It propels us to focus on the kindness in our life and inspires us to spread the kindness to others.

The more we spread the kindness, the more our bounty will increase. This basic truth is simplified in *The Prayer of Jabez: Breaking Through to the Blessed Life* by bestselling author Bruce Wilkinson.

PART 3
Gratitude: Love that Paints Beauty in the Soul

"God is energy. Energy is in everything, Energy cannot be created nor destroyed. It can only be transformed."

Prelude

Still athirst, the awakening traveler asked, "Kind Master, why is God invisible to my brother and me, and to all His people? And where does He live?"

The kind Master smiled, then whispered softly, "My dear child, God is visible everywhere! He lives in your disabled brother, and in you and all His creation!"

Overwhelmed by the response, the awakening traveler fell to her knees in prayers of gratitude and total praise to Eternal God.

1. God Is in Everything and Everything is in God.

Gratitude is the best feeling we could ever have. It is the ultimate joy of living. It is perhaps the genesis of all other really good feelings in the human experiences.

The experiences of gratitude journal writing awaken us to the wisdom that God is the love within us, the love that paints beauty in the soul.

Gratitude is a love that paints beauty in the soul. It is the best feeling we could ever have. Perhaps this is the reason gratitude journaling can easily become a passion. It is filled with the spirit of love, thanksgiving and humility.

As we continue to evolve through gratitude journal writing, we learn from wise disciples like Father Damian, the clergyman for the Veterans Administration Medical Center in Miami, Florida, that "God is energy; and energy cannot be created nor destroyed...just transformed."

Energy is in everything and everything is in energy; God is in everything and everything is in God. God is love; love is energy. The world spins on the energy of love.

As children of God, we are energy; we are love, we are life.

With attitudes of gratitude, we give and receive joy through acts of kindness.

Caregiving experiences enable us to explore the many areas of love when we engage in gratitude journal writing. We view gratitude as a love that paints beauty in the soul because it extends to us the opportunity to cultivate the fruits of the spirit where the energy of love is the major attitude.

Utilizing the prayers energy of gratitude, our lives can be transformed from fear to faith; from loneliness to love; from self-doubt to self-discovery.

Mysteriously, the experience of being a family caregiver and recording the experiences of spiritual, moral and social growth helps us to see how beautifully love is propelling us as we continue to evolve.

Family caregiving modifies attitudes, unlocks the fullness of our hearts and minds through the expression of gratitude, and yields that level of satisfaction and joy which comes from a personal relationship with our Creator.

We must be thankful that gratitude is an expression of love that paints beauty in the soul as we practice the art of living triumphantly. When we practice the art of seeing ourselves in others, we feel the spirit of brotherly love within. With prayerful insight, we posses the energy to extend this feeling of love to all humanity.

When we see ourselves in others, who then can we harm? Adhering to this principle, we humbly and thankfully embrace the spiritual brotherhood of man.

When we embrace the spiritual brotherhood of man, we will realize that this is the only way whereby peace on earth and good will among men can be realized.

Caregivers have a mission to spread the wisdom that comes from caregiving. This wisdom can best be defined under the motif of kindness.

When we define gratitude as a form of love that paints beauty in the soul, we are fully aware that this beauty grows out of harmonious relationships with other people, especially our disabled loved ones. It stems from an attitude of gratitude. It allows us to perform our duties beautifully and with a passion. It enables us to meet the challenges of each day with a spirit of kindness, excerpting from our gratitude journals the spiritual gifts of wisdom obtained.

PART 4
Gratitude: The Soul's Noble Attitude

"Whatsoever you do to the least of my people, that you do unto me." — Matthew 26:40

Prelude

"Kind Master, Jesus of Nazareth taught us by example how to be humble. While caring for my brother, how can I learn to be more humble?"

The kind Master softly answered, "Your brother will teach you, my child. But first, you must be quiet and listen with a noble heart. In the quietness of your soul you must meditate and pray. When you see the spiritual message, share your light with the world of caregivers."

1. Anatomy of a Noble Soul

Today, as I listen to the national news, I am even more aware that caregiving teaches us that there is only one adventure which is more satisfying and joyful than the attempt to discover God's will, and that is the supreme experience of trying our best to obey His divine will.

Jesus of Nazareth, noble, dauntless and brave in his ministry, lived among us to show us by example how to be grateful, how to forgive others and how to love them. "Learn of me for I am meek and humble of heart," he said to us, his brothers.

It was the hope of many of my Christian friends to visit Jesus of Nazareth's birthplace this holy, historical and momentous period 2000-2001, but due to man's inhumanity and selfishness, the beautiful city of Jerusalem is embroiled in a civil war. How strange that this should happen just when the Christian world was joyously awaiting this miraculous and exciting occasion—the advent of a new century.

Christians throughout the world are now folded in prayer, asking God for the spiritual message of this human experience, and to order our steps in His Word as we, the people of the world, accept our spiritual mission to help solve the problems that are triggering this civil war.

Jesus of Nazareth has shown us that we are our brother's keeper. Caregiving experiences teach us how to answer the call of being our brother's keeper and how to follow the teachings of Jesus in order that we might have life and have it abundantly. On the journey of life, caregiving enables us to experience the presence of God in our lives, to religiously adhere to the teachings of Jesus to spread kindness and love, and to see the unity of religion and the Oneness of God.

Christians, the followers of Jesus of Nazareth who is the Christ, make up the largest religious group in the world, numbering more than 840 million. People who are drawn to Jesus love his teachings that we must love God and obey His commandment to love one another. We follow Jesus because he showed us by human example how to love God and obey His commandments to love one another. Jesus showed us by example how to be humble before God, yet great in Him.

Our understanding of Jesus' life is synonymous to my doctoral format, i.e., (1) The Proposal: *tell 'em what you're gonna do; (2) The Dissertation: do it; and (3) The Abstract: show 'em how you did it.*

My husband and I, who enjoy following the teachings of Jesus, refer to this insight as "a format with implications for further study" in spiritual growth.

In our life with multiple sclerosis as caregiver/patient, in which we live with the constant threat of death due to complications, we have found the teachings of Jesus to be the light of life. Jesus' teachings and human examples taught us that pain and death are inevitable but suffering is a choice.

In other words, our perceptions are a choice. We choose what to see, what to believe.

Jesus' life here on earth taught us that greater than life is our personal relationship with God, who commands us to love one another and who awakens us to transcendent wisdom and universal compassion.

"Follow me," Jesus said to us, his brothers and sisters. John and I answered the call with a passion when the universe threw us a lifeline by the name of multiple sclerosis to save us from the disease's disruption and hardship, that we might have life and have it more abundantly. We have entered into His peace and are now joyfully experiencing a life of *thanksliving*. In gratitude, we are sharing the gift by spreading love through acts of kindness. How marvelous to see that an insidious disease could have brought so much grace and love!

The experiences of caregiving taught us that it is, indeed, a spiritual mission that gives us the opportunity to be Christlike in our relationships with our loved ones and with all humanity.

In gratitude to Jesus Christ for his great teachings, Christians all over the world wanted to visit his birthplace and even kiss the ground on which he walked. The civil war in Jerusalem seems to send us a profound message in the words of an old Negro Spiritual: "there's destruction in the land...God's gonna raise His hand... Oh-o-o time is a'winding up. Your time and my time, time is a'winding up..."

And even now as I am engrossed in writing this in the silence of my higher self, echoes from the beautiful anthem, *Jerusalem*, which we used to sing with astounding harmony in the high school choral ensemble softly resound:

"Jerusalem, Jerusalem, O turn thee to the Lord, thy God...O turn, thee, O turn thee, unto to thy God..."

Because God answers the soul's attitude, we must ask Him to please hear our prayers when we, as a united people on planet earth, pray from the depths of our hearts the song written by Sy Miller and Jill Jackson, *Let There Be Peace on Earth.* Let us, with a passion, embrace its powerful lyrics:

"...Let there be peace on earth, a peace that was meant to be... With God as our Father, brothers all are we... let us walk with each other in perfect harmony. ...With every breath I take, let this be my solemn vow... to take each moment and live each moment in peace eternally... Let there be peace on earth and let it begin with me."

May God answer our soul's attitude, for Jesus of Nazareth has shown us by human example that "gratitude is the mark of a noble soul."

2. The Power of Love vs The Love of Power

On this October 9, 2000, we thank Eternal God for loving us all unconditionally even amid the new Mideast bloodshed in Jerusalem, The Holy Land, as Israeli-Palestinian violence move into its tenth day. Because we are our brother's keeper and are commanded to love one another, we pray that Israel will implement international resolutions about Jerusalem's status to guarantee that freedom of religion for Christians, Muslims and Jews is respected within the city. We are grateful for Pope John Paul II who stated that: "The Holy Land must be the land of peace and fraternity. That is what God wants."

Wisdom teaches us that when the power of love replaces the love of power we will be Christ-like in our peaceful relationship with each other. In gratitude to God for His son, Jesus, who taught us by example how to love, each of us as individuals needs to *always* silently and meditatively pray:

"Dear Lord, please teach me only one thing; how to love the world the way you love me."

We must pray that the Creator will help us, as a people united, to awaken and to return to love with an attitude of gratitude so that we can hear the spiritual message of this human experience and, in gratitude, adhere to its teachings.

Awakening to divine love is a mystery to us humans who are aware that life is a mystery to be lived, and a series of problem solving situations. We are thankful to the universe for teaching us through human experiences that **Love** is the essence of life, that *kindness* is the truest religion, and for revealing to us that our mission here on earth is to live in love and service that will help promote social justice, universal peace and brotherly love.

We are thankful to our Creator also for teaching us through life's experiences that the wisdom of love is born in suffering just as His son, Jesus of Nazareth...God Incarnate, has shown us. He showed us by myriad examples and by the use of parables that the way we treat other people is the way we treat our personal God.

We are grateful to Jesus of Nazareth for teaching us the wisdom and joy of living a life of gratitude.

We are grateful to Him for teaching us the joy of loving God, of loving others, and the beauty of forgiving one another.

We are grateful to Him for awakening us to the wisdom, joy and abundant blessings of being thankful and kind.

We are grateful to him for showing, even amid the calm and the strife, that gratitude is the mark of a truly noble soul.

Jesus of Nazareth is indeed a truly noble soul. We have a passion for studying his life because we, too, want to be noble souls. We want to follow his example of living a life of kindness and compassion, and enter into his joy of loving and serving God.

Jesus of Nazareth showed us how to obey God's commandments that we love one another even amid the calm and the strife of human experiences, of turmoil and bloodshed. Obeying God's commandments to love one another gives us the joy of *feeling* the love for one another and the peace and joy of eternal life.

"I am come that they might have life, and that they might have it more abundantly." —John 10:10

Gratitude journal writing, in conjunction with my study of Jesus, has taught me that if we want to be abundantly blessed by Eternal God, we need to pray from the depths of the soul and have unshrinking faith in Him. We must have faith even amid the calm and the strife. We learn that prayers of gratitude and gratitude journaling are like the obverse and reverse of the same coin. In journaling as in meditation and prayer, we remain in soulful silence.

PART 5

Gratitude amid The Calm and the Strife

The most beautiful and humble prayer is a sincere 'thank you' raised to heaven in the spirit of love, kindness and humility amid adversity. — Father Damian

Prelude

The humbled, awakening traveler lifted her hands in prayer and asked, "Kind Master, how can I best express my gratitude to you for the calm and strife of caregiving?"

"My dear child," the kind master whispered softly, "Let your words of prayer flow from the depths of your heart."

"I Lift My Hands in Total Praise to You."

Eternal Father, inasmuch as the emergence of self is a continuous event of evolution, we gratefully accept the theory that "we humans never arrive; we are always arriving."

I found this to be a basic truth while documenting my life experiences in a series of gratitude journals suggested by your messenger, Oprah Winfrey. Help us to live a life of gratitude to You even amid the calm and strife of our evolving souls.

Just as we love, respect and appreciate your religious ministers who teach us of your kindness, we love, respect and appreciate Oprah because she shares her love for You with us, her listeners, who thirst for your spirit of kindness and compassion. Her ministry is indeed your blessing to those of us who listen to her wisdom. She awakens us to the joy of remembering our spirit and recording our gratitude in a journal.

Performing this task has become a personal spiritual experience which teaches us that attitude is indeed everything. And that an attitude of gratitude awakens us to the genuine kindness, love and compassion of others and helps us to return to our natural state of joyfulness. In remembering our spirit of love which you planted within us, we are able to bestow this spirit of love upon our fellow man. Love is the desire to do good to others.

In recording my life's lessons in an endeavor to cope with the turmoil of family caregiving, I realized that I was always being awakened to higher stages of love, compassion and gratitude that stemmed from higher levels of wisdom, knowledge and understanding. In quietness and after following the continuous quenching of thirst, I am always arriving to another level of thirst.

Writing in my series of gratitude journals enabled me to recall the many, many times You, through your earthly angels throughout the world and in nursing facilities, have responded to my cry for help and understanding...showing me that the most important duty in life is "people giving of themselves in love and service to one another." It is You who give them the gift to give.

Seeing this lesson in action as my mind flashed into the past, present and future of my existence, I felt the spirit of love within urging me to keep writing and let the spiritual messages unfold, amid tears of gratitude.

2. Letting Gratitude Become a Way of Life

As we are broken open by our experiences, we begin to be grateful for what is, and if we live long enough and authentically enough, gratitude becomes a way of life.
Mark Nepo

Eternal God, it has been said that making the best of an apparently bad situation is a sign of creativity. Discovering this was total joy as I, with the help of many of your vessels of love, evolved in spite of adversity by adhering to the principle: "We spiritual beings can be nowhere except in the mind of God."

Through your guidance, family caregiving has taught me to view all life's experiences in the context of a loving plan.

Therefore, when I viewed my husband's chronic illness, multiple sclerosis (usually called MS), and my experiences in the context of a loving plan, that view constituted the greatest source of spiritual support imaginable. I saw your vessels of love, through whom You speak, in every walk of life. This feeling of gratitude and joy overwhelms me.

So overwhelming was this continuous awakening, my husband and I ventured into a world of creative writing, expressing the joy, love, respect and appreciation to the host of earthly angels You sent to help us on this journey. Thank You for this direct line of creation from You through us to other family caregivers and their disabled loved ones.

Our gratitude has become a way of life. The feeling of gratitude is like awakening to a new world filled with glowing sunlight.

As we continue to awaken, we see the interconnectedness, interdependence, and interrelatedness of our existence in the material world of commodities and services. Viewing our world from the perspective of gratitude, we see the roots of our human happiness in the beautiful context of your Divine plan. We see everything as holy.

Our lifelong battle with multiple sclerosis was a gift that led us to the joy of returning to You and experiencing that You are indeed our natural state of joyfulness.

It has been said that a search for God is a search for self. In our humble search for You to help us cope with our adversity, we found ourselves as we wrote about these experiences and as You, in our cry for help, revealed their spiritual messages to us. Thank You for speaking to all of us through our daily human experiences. Thank You for giving us the wisdom to silently listen. *Ye that have ears, let them hear. —Matthew 11:15*

We saw the beauty of your kingdom, people engaged in their various jobs helping people in the spirit of kindness as they continue to unlock their Divine inheritance. Gratitude journaling has taught us that our various jobs are a direct line of creation, from You through us to all mankind. We are most grateful for the writer, Witness Lee, who tells us that "All fullness of the Father is in the Son; all that is in the Son is in the spirit, and all that is in the spirit is in the man. This is the very Savior in whom we believe. This is the very Lord whom we serve. This is the very God whom we worship. This is the Christ who dwells in us as our life."

Throughout our gratitude journaling, You have shown us the wisdom of loving, respecting and appreciating others, and that their kindnesses are symbols of your love—a love that is a direct line of creation from You, through us humans, to all humanity.

PART 6
Gratitude: The Symbols of Love

We should not look for why the suffering comes,
but for what the suffering can teach us.
— Father Raymond Crowe.

Prelude

The newly awakening traveler is overwhelmed with joy that multiple sclerosis, sometimes called MS and Mysterious Stranger, is seen in the context of a loving plan. She continues in prayer; knowing that to her, MS also means "My Savior!"

In quietness, the kind Master tenderly whispers into her silence, "My child, MS also means 'My Spirit' that dwells in you, your loved one and his multiple sclerosis. All *creation* is holy."

Hearing His silent voice and feeling His presence within, joy flooded her soul.

1. Suffering is a Spiritual Teacher

Eternal Father, it was through your divine guidance that my husband and I wrote our first book, *Mysterious Stranger Aboard*, a euphemism for MS Aboard that chronicled our (then) 40-year battle with multiple sclerosis.

Writing the book changed my life spiritually and dramatically because I realized that when I was talking with my higher self, your spirit of wisdom was present, revealing an interpretation of my human experiences. The spiritual message accompanying each experience was clear and softly revealed.

On bent knees amid stifling tears, I humbly asked You a similar question formerly asked by a brother: "Heavenly Father, why are there so many suffering people in the world like my chronically ill, beloved husband and all these disabled war veterans?" Your answer came to me in a soft whisper: "They are here to scientifically teach you, my child, how to love and care for one another as I love and care for you."

I thank You for this spiritual awakening as I now realize that man is a subject for religion and science, and that all life's teachings are branches of science. Religion is a science. We are here to help each other in love and service, learning and teaching in the spirit of gratitude as we experience life.

This loving plan with its spiritual agenda awakens us to man's interrelatedness, interdependence, and interconnectedness.

The experiences of family caregiving and gratitude journaling have shown me this basic truth of people helping people in the spirit of love and service.

When we read about the lives of the many spiritual role models who have gone through some of the most devastating tragedies imaginable and those who have to live every day with the fact that they are physically disabled, we are amazed how they have turned their tragedies into blessings.

Pain comes to teach us, and if we become chronically depressed to the point that we cannot pray a silent "Thank You," we've lost the spiritual lesson. When we see pain as having a purpose in our life, it steers us closer to our life's mission.

Before my husband was diagnosed with multiple sclerosis, we were looking for a way to make a living. Since his chronic illness, we have been looking for ways to make a contribution to help uplift humanity. Gratitude journaling has shown us the many symbols of love, people helping people throughout the world. Utilizing this insight, we be became "playwrights for the children" and began writing and producing a series of musical docudramas that highlight the lives of outstanding role models who have triumphed over adversity. Thousands of school students attend our productions that emphasize multicultural education and literacy. In addition, we are writing and producing inspirational books on family caregiving, portraying the experience as a spiritual mission to spread love and service to others.

Hospitals and nursing homes are learning institutions that teach us by human examples a world of symbols of love where love is international. Every employee from sanitation engineers to medical professionals show us, by example, how their services fit into the context of Your divine plan.

People need people. People need commodities and services. People, in rendering these commodities and services, are symbols of love. It does not necessarily matter whether or not they recognize their performances as symbols of love, but it would help them to know that this kind service is a direct line of creation, from You through us as individuals to humankind.

Attitudes of Gratitude are symbols of love in which we glorify You through our services to one another.

Gratitude journaling reveals to us these symbols of love, and the more grateful we are for the symbols of love we give and receive, the more our bounty increases.

As retired school teachers who now are writers/producers, my husband and I are grateful to You for making our lives abundantly productive. With your blessings, we have been able to establish endowed scholarships at several colleges and universities of our choice, and make numerous contributions, including massive hours of voluntary services, to a variety of charities.

Attitudes of gratitude in everyday living have taught us that the spirit of being thankful alights our inner world with unspeakable joy.

Eternal Father, thank you for showing us that gratitude

gives birth to happiness, and that attitudes of gratitude are indeed symbols of Your love.

PART 7

Gratitude: The Spirit of Kindness and Concern

And he said unto me, "My grace is sufficient for thee;
for my strength is made perfect in weakness."
Most gladly, therefore, will I rather glory in my infirmities,
that the power of Christ may rest upon me.
—2 Corinthians 12-9

Prelude

And then, feeling the presence of God in all creation, the traveler's spirit humbly asked, "O, Divine Master, how can I best express my sincere gratitude to you for responding to our prayers that flowed from the pages of our gratitude journals?"

The Master silently whispered, "Again, my dear child, you must be still and listen to the meditations of your heart. Then, feel your love for Me within, and let your words flow freely."

1. Human Experiences are Miracle Gifts

Eternal God, You have revealed to us through our gratitude journaling that spiritual awareness is a sense of gratitude for the life within and that, especially amid adversity, love finds expression through kindness and concern.

You have shown us through human experiences that possessing an attitude of gratitude is the key that unlocks the life within, around and beyond us. It extends to us the gifts of abundant spiritual and economic joy, and unshrinking faith.

As a family caregiver, I fervently thank You for this experience and for the wisdom learned through gratitude journal writing.

Gratitude journaling awakens us to the awareness that our everyday life experiences show us by human examples that love always finds expression through kindness and concern toward one another. Being fully cognizant to this basic truth is indeed a blessing from You to us. According to Your Word spoken through Reverend Dr. Barbara King to us, it focuses the following three powerful secrets of a peaceful and happy life:

1. In all things give thanks.
2. Judge not and you will not be judged.
3. Forgive, and you will be forgiven.

Being grateful at all times is not always an easy attitude to possess. But it is in those times of adversity, Eternal Father, when we feel least thankful, that we are most in need of what gratitude can give us, namely:

- Insight for the life within us
- Insight to the life around us, and
- Insight to the life beyond us.

This is why gratitude journaling is a spiritual awakening of the soul.

Wrestling with the chronic illness and following Your divine guidance, my husband and I learned that spiritual awareness opens our eyes to see that the universe is kind. Perceiving this attitude gives us a spirit of gratitude for the life within, around and beyond us. We learned that being our brother's keeper humanizes us all, enabling us to see ourselves in others.

We were made aware that sheer suffering does not teach. Because, if suffering alone taught, all the world would be wise, since everyone suffers. It is Your spirit of love within, around and beyond us that teaches. We listen to You in the silence of our soul's attitude.

That is why we began to search for the spiritual message

of our battle with multiple sclerosis, inasmuch as we firmly believe that You speak to us all through our human, everyday experiences.

As a result of our belief, we were able to view our caregiving experiences with the chronic illness in the context of Your loving plan to teach us the wisdom of love and compassion, and to share with humanity Your message that love always finds expression through kindness and concern toward one another.

2. Human Experiences are Expressions of Divine Love

> *"As an elect of God, holy and beloved, put on tender mercies, kindness, humility, meekness, longsuffering; bearing with one another, and forgiving one another."*
> *—Colossians 3:12-13*

We are truly grateful that, through your continued guidance, our experiences as patient and family caregiver, beautifully taught us that **love** is the "mysterious stranger aboard" our lives and, in the spirit of gratitude, it is shown through acts of kindness and concern.

In our gratitude journal writing, the myriad caregiving experiences You gave us awakened us to an awareness that gratitude is love in action, and that:

(1) *Love paints beauty in the soul.*
(2) Love's wisdom should always be our guide amid t*he calm and the strife.*
(3) Kind services from others are *symbols of love* for which we should be grateful and say "thank you."
(4) Love can create within us an *attitude of gratitude.*
(5) *Love finds expression through kindness and concern.*

(6) *Caring for the caregiver* is a symbol of love's wisdom and gratitude.
(7) By cultivating a spirit of kindness, love and gratitude, *we create our own happiness.*
(8) Love teaches us the joy of *touching hearts, lifting spirits.*
(9) Love's wisdom teaches us that *gratitude is the mother of human happiness.*

Enjoying this direct line of creation from You through us to our readers, my husband and I have ventured into a writing spree that seems unending. Thank you for granting us the gift of experiencing a life of creativity to enhance moral and spiritual support and growth for ourselves and for other patients/caregivers whose lives are plagued with adversity.

3. Adversity is a Divine Blessing

I have been led to understand, Eternal Father, why adversity is a blessing because through your teachings, suffering enabled my husband and me to strengthen our spiritual lives by following the lessons of Jesus of Nazareth as well as learn from the suffering experiences of our biblical character, Job. They taught us that adversity offers us the gift of unshrinking faith in You with a love that surpasses all understanding. What a gift!

In following the wisdom learned from Scripture, we both were also able to cultivate the spirit of gratitude as wisely suggested by one of your disciples, Oprah Winfrey. We discovered that gratitude journaling is a pathway to Your spirit within us.

Under Oprah's motif, "Remembering Your Spirit," John and I were swept into the mystery and beauty of Your love, making each day a day of thanksgiving. And the November

2000, issue of her national magazine, "O", celebrates the art of gratitude, urging us readers to give ourselves the gift of gratitude.

We thank You for your world of earthly angels like Oprah and others who share your wisdom with us, and who use their gifts to help give us all spiritual support on life's journey.

Utilizing the wisdom of your loving plan which journaling unlocked, we were able to overcome the strains, stress and tensions of multiple sclerosis which we felt between ourselves and our surroundings. In developing the art of appreciation, we experienced the gift of joy and serenity in our lives, and we now feel as one in the heart of all humanity. We were awakened to an understanding that our mission in life is to love and to serve humanity. Help us to always stay focused on this divine mission, because in so doing, we feel the joy of your spirit that consumes us.

We thank You for awakening us to your spirit of love that lives within us all.

We thank You for teaching us, through human experiences and via your disciples, the wisdom and joy of being grateful as we tap the treasures of appreciative living hidden in our past and present experiences. We thank You for the gifts of caregiving that awaken us to the wisdom that love finds expression through kindness and concern, and that this wisdom must be a major priority in caring for the caregiver, the care recipient and others throughout the world.

Heavenly Father, may we always humbly express our love, gratitude and praise to you. May we always be aware that every work we perform is a direct line of creation from you through us to humanity. We ask this through our Lord Jesus Christ, your Son, who lives and reigns with you, for ever and ever. Amen.

PART 8

Gratitude: The Spirit of Caring for the Caregiver

"I am only afraid that at the same time the world will have turned into one large hospital where everyone is everybody else's humane nurse."—Goethe

Prelude

Finally experiencing the joy of inner peace, the awakening traveler asked? "Kind Master, how can I hold on to this feeling of peacefulness on a daily basis as I continue my tremendous spiritual mission of caring for my loved one?"

The Master softly whispered, "My child, try to follow, religiously, the lessons taught by your loved one on how to take care of your health. When you learn to practice extreme self-care, your loved one will benefit. When you awaken to the spiritual message, write from your world of family caregiving and share your light with others."

1. Gratitude and the Caregiver

One of the major lessons learned from gratitude journaling and from caregiving experiences is that when we change our thoughts, feelings and attitudes, our outer experiences will change automatically. We become transformed and we live a life of thanksgiving. Inside ourselves or outside, we never have to change what we see, only the way we see it.

If we want to continue to give care, it is essential that we look after ourselves. Many family caregivers suffer serious health problems as the result of excessive and stressful demands on them of looking after their loved ones or friends. If caregivers fail to look after themselves, the world will evolve into one large hospital where everybody is everybody else's caregiver.

Gratitude journal writing experiences show us by daily examples that an attitude of gratitude promotes good physical, mental and economic health.
In addition...

- An attitude of gratitude makes us feel happy.
- An attitude of gratitude unlocks the fullness of our spiritual life, enabling us to be kind and compassionate toward others.
- An attitude of gratitude turns what we have into enough and more.
- An attitude of gratitude helps us to understand that no one belongs to us except in memory, releasing us from being control freaks.
- An attitude of gratitude transforms our lives, gives us the gift of humility and an unshrinkable faith in Eternal God.
- An attitude of gratitude connects us to spirit, filling our hearts with love, respect and appreciation for ourselves and for others.

2. Caregiving Strategies

In order to be effective in taking on the responsibility of being a caregiver, we need to be aware of the following strategies:

- Learn as much as possible about managing stress in order to avoid caregiver burnout.
- Learn to master the art of meditation and cultivate an attitude of gratitude. These experiences will help you clear the pathway to your higher self, where you will find answers to help you on life's journey.
- Try to view family caregiving as a spiritual mission. When you perceive caregiving in the context of a loving

plan, that constitutes the highest spiritual support imaginable.
- Be familiar with the four stages of caregiver burnout so that you can avoid being a victim.

3. Jobs Caregivers Can Share

While it is true that sickness and infirmity of a loved one can also take its toll on you as a caregiver, the following list of additional services might be considered on pacing yourself as a family caregiver, knowing how and when to seek more help, and conserving your energy to preserve your own physical and emotional health.

- Give a haircut
- Make an ice cream sundae
- Do the laundry
- Give the dog a bath
- Take out the garbage
- Water the garden/flowers
- Give a manicure/pedicure
- Cut the grass
- Dust
- Give primary caregiver a break
- Cook a meal
- Write "thank you" notes/cards
- Take the patient for a drive
- Compliment another caregiver
- Feed the pets
- Take kids to doctor/dentist
- Balance the checkbook
- Play soothing music
- Change the sheets
- Program the VCR
- Rent some videos

- Take kids out for recreation
- Give a massage
- Help with cosmetics
- Write cards/letters for patient
- Clean eyeglasses
- Give a birthday party for child
- Clean the bathroom
- Bring fresh flowers
- Make a fruit salad/smoothie
- Write/share a poem
- Go to the pharmacy
- Write a letter for patient
- Help fill out insurance forms
- Buy postage stamps
- Clean the bird cage
- Visit in the hospital
- Make collage of photos
- Go to post office
- Walk the dog
- Give a back rub
- Bake a cake
- Get the newspaper
- Help child with homework
- Vacuum the house
- Put up new curtains
- Do the ironing
- Take patient for an outing
- Help with a bath
- Find someone to do the taxes
- Water the plants
- Return videos
- Return books to library
- Fix the clocks to correct time

4. *Plan for the Future*

As soon as you begin caring for your loved one or friend, you need to plan for the immediate future and consider what is ahead for both of you. In your plans, try to include family members and the loved one, if possible.

There will perhaps come a time when it is impossible for you to provide care in your home. The care recipient may need long-term care or a nursing home placement. As a caregiver, you should not view this need as a sign of failure. Instead, see it as a chapter in the progression of the illness. In either facility and with gratitude, you can still visit and give quality time and moral support with kindness, love and compassion.

You are very important, and what you do is very important. Make a special effort to take good care of yourself.

PART 9

Gratitude: The Art of Creating Our Own Happiness

Where is the spiritual, childlike-life of gratitude we have lost in living? —Father Damian

Prelude

"Kind Master, how can my ailing brother teach me the art of creating my own happiness?" the awakening traveler asked?

The Master softly replied, "If you will sit quietly, listen and meditate, my child, he will share this knowledge with you through gratitude journal writing. You will pray for understanding and my light will shine within you. Light your candle and share your awakening with the world of family caregivers."

1. Awakening the Childlike Attitude Within Us

For many of us, it is interesting to reflect on our childhood and realize that "before we can count, we are taught to be grateful for what others do." With this feeling of gratitude, we create our own happiness. And then as we reflect on our adulthood, we begin to ask ourselves, "Where is the spiritual, childlike-life of gratitude we have lost in living?"

One of the miracle gifts of gratitude journal writing is that it enables us to look within ourselves and find the child we lost in living, because the experience is a program of self-discovery and spiritual psychotherapy. It tears away the inflated ego.

Gratitude journal writing shows us by human experiences that:

- We create our own happiness by possessing an attitude of gratitude.
- We create our own happiness by treating others as we wish to be treated.

- We create our own happiness by loving the God within us and obeying His Will to love one another in the spirit of kindness and service.
- We create our own happiness by embracing the child-like spirit of gratitude and humility within us.
- We create our own happiness by silently praying from the depths of the heart, in the spirit of humility and unconditional love: "Let Thy Will be done."

But because of our busy schedules that keep us flooded with anxieties and tensions, we sometimes fail to take time, see and appreciate the importance of knowing that we already posses the tools for creating our own happiness. They were given us as a gift from our Creator. When we accept the wisdom that we humans are interrelated, interdependent and interconnected, we will realize that the Creator has given us the key that unlocks the doors to our inherited state of happiness.

The experience of caregiving is one of the major keys that unlocks the doors of happiness, through gratitude journal writing.

But, many of us are unwilling to engage in a program of gratitude journal writing or to even regularly meditate or pray because we feel that these "Know-Thyself" programs of spiritual psychotherapy for one's self are too time consuming.

Human experiences have taught us that there are numerous tried and true ways to overcome the strains and tensions we feel between ourselves and our surroundings. One of those ways is to silently meditate, and Divine Intelligence will reveal the answers. Fortunately, one of the major miracles of gratitude journal writing is that it is a program of silent meditation in which we communicate with Divine Intelligence.

There is an adage that says: "We would have inner peace, if we would look within." Unfortunately, many of us have an outside world that is far too noisy to let us stop and look within our inside world.

Divine Intelligence has shown us that we can regain the spirit of joy and serenity by locking ourselves in the mystery of love. When we cultivate the art of being appreciative, we gain a sense of life's meaning and purpose. Thus, we discover that the kingdom of heaven is within us. With this revelation, we become like little children.

Our brother, Jesus of Nazareth, has said to us:
"Suffer little children to come unto me,
and forbid them not, for such is the
kingdom of heaven." — (Matt. 19:14).

With an attitude of gratitude for this spiritual lesson, we should meditate and ask Eternal God to help us find the child within us so that we can, with humility and gratitude, enter the kingdom of heaven.

2. *The Journey Within to our inner child*

The real self is the love within us. It is the child of God."
—Father Damian

Wisdom teaches us that in every life there is a child's spirit within us which does not answer to the question "why", but is a loving spirit which we must embrace, no matter how it behaves.

We are told that it is a spirit that is joyful and sorrowful, beautiful and enriching, a symbol of love, yet we must remember that it is always for us. It is never against us.

This spirit is an eternal child, a symbol of love, something that is always becoming, is never completed, and calls for unceasing care, attention, and education. This is the spiritual part of the human personality which wants to develop and become whole.

Veterans Administration Medical Center's Catholic priest, Father Damian, has taught us that when we exercise the child within, it brings us into the world. We are all here to live out the child's destiny. We are told that the child is person to the whole person. Each child's life is a fresh experiment in humankind's spiritual evolution. It represents a wholeness which embraces the very depths of nature. The child is our true spirit with its inherited divinity waiting to be unlocked. Inasmuch as we still see the Christ Child in the Lord Jesus, we need to always see the "Christlike child" in each other.

We grown-ups are grateful to realize that it takes a long time to become like a child, and should gratefully awaken to the wisdom that it is never too late to have a happy childhood. How often do we see the soul-touching lyrics of meaningful songs of childhood and forget to thank the Creator for the author who wrote them. Usually they are written with such depths and feelings that our hearts overflow with joy.

Reflecting on this and all the many teachings of spiritual leaders throughout the world who have shared with us their wisdom, I am reminded of a joyful song of gratitude from my childhood. It is a song which my younger sister, Earline, and I would often sing at home, at church and at school.

A PRAYER OF GRATITUDE
(Author Unknown)

(Verse one)
Can a little child like me
Thank Our Father faithfully?

Yes, oh yes, be good and true,
Faithful, kind in all you do;
Love the Lord and do your part
Learn to say with all your heart...

(Chorus)
"Father, we thank Thee
"Father we thank Thee
"Father in heaven we than-n-n-nk Thee.

(Verse Two)
"For the fruits upon the tree
"For the birds that sing of Thee
"For Your love and tender care
"For Your children everywhere
"For a life so filled with love
"For the sun that shines above."
(Repeat Chorus)

Thank you, Eternal Father, for parents who knew You and your divine love for all of us, your children throughout the world. Help us to always see each other as symbols of love so that we can, in our efforts to obey your divine will to be kind to one another. Amen.

In addition to the song, I am reminded of another prayer of gratitude our loving parents eagerly taught us all when we were little children. I was told that we were taught this prayer even before we could count. It is a prayer we always said before bedtime and upon arising. When I was a primary and elementary school teacher, I taught it to my students and it was a major part of our morning devotion:

THANK YOU, GOD
(Author Unknown)

"Thank You for the world so sweet
Thank You for the food we eat
Thank You for the birds that sing
Thank You, God, for everything!" - Amen.

The following is a prayer of gratitude which my younger sister taught me when we were little children. Her kindergarten teacher had taught it to her students and they recited it every morning during their devotional exercises. Years later, when I was a teacher, I gladly taught it to my students and they loved reciting it every morning before beginning class.

THANK YOU
(Author Unknown)

Now before we work today
Let us not forget to pray
That God has kept us through the night
And brought us to the morning light.
Help us, Lord, to love Thee more
Than we've ever done before
In our work and in our play
Be Thou with us everyday
For Jesus' sake, Amen.

3. Precious Memories via Gratitude Journaling

While it is true that no one belongs to us except in memory, how sadly I recall my little 8-year old student, David, who used to love reciting the prayer, "Thank You" and how he was struck and killed by an automobile as he was riding his bicycle on his neighborhood street. I recall the touching funeral service and the unceasing tears of his father, mother, siblings and classmates. I especially remember how, immediately following the service, his young parents thanked me over and over again for the love, kindness and compassion I had shown their little child who loved the prayers and songs I had taught him about love. They told me how excitedly he taught them to his siblings and how they enjoyed sharing them with their playmates and Sunday School classes. I told the parents that their little boy had enriched my spiritual life by giving me the opportunity to be connected with his spirit, and that we are all one in the Spirit of love.

Astounded, I now ask my higher self, "Lord, if we can always see the child in Jesus of Nazareth, why can't we always see the child in each other? His life here on earth set the perfect example for us to follow."

Even as I write this episode, it seems I can hear David's childlike voice singing proudly and drowning out his fellow classmates:

THE GOLDEN KEYS
(Author Unknown)

"Good Morning!" That's the golden key
That unlocks everyday for me
All through the day I use the keys
of "Thank You," "Pardon Me" and "Please."

THE GOOD MORNING SONG
(Author Unknown)

Good Morning, Good Morning, Good morning to you
To teachers and classmates, oh how do you do?
Good morning to you! Good morning to you!
We're all in our places, with sun shiny faces
For this is the way to start a new day.

"And the new day is_ (write in the specific day)," I would softly say to the energetic class immediately following the song and pointing to the blackboard with chalk in hand. David was always quick in leading the appropriate litany of responses (i.e.," Today is Monday, November 11, 1972. The weather is sunny, etc.). Thus, we would write our fine-line news and afterwards, read it in unison.

It has been said that teachers teach the way they were taught. Fortunately, when I was in school, we were always taught the art of cultivating love, compassion and gratitude.

And as I now write, I recall the following song of gratitude my sister, Earline, and I learned from our family. We would often sing it together and with classmates while in primary school and Sunday School. Joyfully, I had taught the song to my students when, years later, I became a school teacher. This, too, was one of David's favorite songs. His words were always clear and pronounced with feelings of childlike love.

FATHER, WE THANK THEE
(Author Unknown)

Father, we thank Thee for the night
And for the pleasant morning light
For rest and food and loving care

And all that makes the world so fair.
Help us to do the things we should
To be to others kind and good
In all we do, in work or play
To grow more loving every day.

Eternal Father, thank You for restoring, through caregiving experiences and gratitude journal writing, the happy life of gratitude I had lost in living. Please awaken today's children, of the twenty-first century, to the spiritual gift of gratitude; and awaken the adult world of leaders to listen to our children's cry for spiritual help. Teaching children to be grateful is a priority. But, how can we teach that which we ourselves do not practice? Please, help us to awaken to the spiritual need of daily expressing gratitude to you. Amen.

4. The Healing Power of Gratitude Journal Writing

The November 2000, issue of "*O,*" The Oprah Magazine, tells us that "One single *grateful thought* raised to heaven is the most perfect prayer," and that gratitude has a cleansing effect on the soul; healing from the inside out. To say "Thank You" is an act of spiritual power. Oprah's magazine clearly emphasizes that if the only *prayer* you ever say in your whole life is *"Thank You,"* that alone would indeed be enough.

When it comes to expressing gratitude through creative writing, the written word is like oceans of prayers. Writing in a gratitude journal heals us from the inside out. We come face to face with our true selves...the "I " that is "me."

The lessons learned by gratitude journal writing reveal to us that when we truly live from a grateful heart, we experience the best feeling we could ever have. Living from a grateful heart is an attitude. We know from life's teachings that attitude is everything and we need to teach our young generation this basic truth. We need to keep emphasizing to them that ingratitude makes us very unhappy. Most anger and feelings of emptiness, disconnectedness and depressions stem from feelings of ingratitude.

Human experiences have taught us that when we look to others for fulfillment, we will never be fulfilled. When our spirit of happiness depends on money, we can never be happy with ourselves. If we expect someone or something outside ourselves to make us happy, we lose our power to choose...to create our own happiness. But, when we form the habit of touching lives and lifting spirits, we experience a state of happiness that gives us the kind of inner peace we all seek.

5. The Cry of The Future Generation

The following poem, which I found on the Internet and revised, tells the sad story of how we are denying today's children the joy of cultivating the spirit of love. It is a cry for help...a cry for moral and spiritual values.

THE NEW SCHOOL PRAYER
FOR THE NEW MILLENNIUM
(Author unknown)

Now I sit me down in school
Where praying is against the rule;
For this great nation under God
Finds mention of Him very odd.

If Scripture now the class recites
It violates the Bill of Rights.
And every time my head I bow
Becomes a federal matter now.
Our hair can be purple or orange or green;

That's no offense, it's the freedom scene.
The law is specific, the law is precise;
Prayers spoken aloud is a serious vice.

For praying in a public hall
Might offend someone with no faith at all.
In silence alone we must meditate,
God's name is prohibited by the State.

We're allowed to cuss and dress like freaks;
And pierce our noses, tongues and cheeks.
They've outlawed guns; but first the Bible;
To quote the Good Book makes me liable.

We can elect a pregnant (Senior) Queen,
And the unwed dad, our King, we've seen.
We can get our condoms and birth controls,
Study witchcraft, vampires and totem poles.

We can abort the unborn child
By butchering it the doctors' style;
And many schools support this choice
Those who oppose don't have a voice.

The Ten Commandments are not allowed,
No "Word of God" must reach this crowd.
It's scary here, I must confess,
When chaos reigns the school's a mess.

So, Lord, this silent plea I make:
Should I be shot, ***my soul please take.***

We have to reinform our adult leaders that prayer is always the solution to society's problems and we need to bring prayers back into our homes, communities and public schools, especially prayers of gratitude that teach moral and spiritual values.

PART 10
Gratitude: The Joy of Being a Candlelight for the World

"He is not heavy; he is my brother."

Prelude

Massaging her forehead, the yet awakening traveler finally asked, "Kind Master, how can my brother teach me to recognize what basically is my mission?"

"My dear child," the Master tenderly answered, "your disabled brother will teach you how to search for self. Then you will see that you are here to be a candlelight to touch lives and lift spirits. But first, you must be quiet, listen attentively and silently meditate daily on your personal experiences and their spiritual messages. Then share your light with others who wish to transform the world through deeds of love and mercy."

1. A Search for Self is a Search for God

Seek for yourself, O man; search for your own true self.
He who seeks shall find—but marvel and joy, he will not
find himself he will find God, or, if he finds himself,
he will find himself in God.
—St. Augustine.

In my world of family caregiving, I was determined to keep my life of caring for my husband from getting in the way of my spiritual well-being. This is why I used the experiences to enhance my spiritual growth by connecting with my inner wisdom to create a personal practice. Through meditation and prayer, I found the glowing light within me. With continuous meditation and gratitude journal writing, I was awakened to the knowledge that the *light* is my divine inheritance, and it is inside me to anoint my soul. But life taught me that this could only be done through experiences of caring for my disabled husband who was sent to teach me and the world how to *feel and live* God's treasury of virtues. Yes, we are called to touch lives and lift spirits as we experience life. We are called to be candlelights for the world. This gift is our inheritance, and it is a choice. John and I made it our choice, and the choice itself is our spiritual blessing and abundance.

By being our brother's keeper, we can become candlelights. As candlelights for the world, we can touch lives and lift spirits.

When we touch lives and lift spirits, we are responding to a call from Eternal God in gratitude for His love and kindness to us.

The wisdom gained from gratitude journal writing reveals to us that the quickest, easiest way to connect to Eternal God is to express our gratitude.

This is because gratitude is the response to the giver of a gift. And when we give thanks for things beyond the gifts we receive from other people, we are thanking the Greater Power for what we have received...symbols of His love.

In helping others, we find God. This truth is reiterated in the following quotation: *I sought my God and he withdrew from me; I sought my soul and it eluded me; I sought my brother, in him I found all three.*

Family caregiving gives the caregiver an opportunity to touch lives and lift spirits through acts of kindness to our disabled brothers. Caregiving is a mission that can test every fiber of the soul because it puts your attitude to a spiritual test. Therefore you need to search for your "self" by frequently praying and mediating in silence. This is an excellent time to communicate with your higher self and feel the spirit of love within. And in your search for inner peace, this is an excellent time to silently whisper in the spirit of love, gratitude and humility, the soul's most humble prayer: "Let Thy Will be done."

When we search for our selves through silent prayer and daily meditation, and if we are lucky to find our selves, we find ourselves in God and we find that God dwells in us. What a miracle! What a joy! What a gift!

Realizing this, we cannot help but make gratitude our daily life of meditation. We cannot help but feel the joy of touching the lives and lifting the spirits of others in need.

Caregiving gives us an opportunity to let gratitude quietly and softly enter our hearts. One of the best ways to approach this decision is to keep a gratitude journal, because writing in our gratitude journal is a silent and humble awakening while communicating with God. When we awake to self, we understand God-flowing in and through us.

When we view caregiving in the spirit of touching lives and lifting spirits, we are grateful and happy that we can be of help to our disabled loved ones and that we are doing the Will of God. With this attitude of gratitude, we experience the joy of inner peace.

2. *The Journey of the Soul*

Touching lives and lifting spirits is a journey of the soul. It is a journey that begins when we dedicate our lives to help others, in gratitude for the help we have received from others.

Consciously cultivating the spirit of thankfulness is a journey of the soul, one that begins when we look around and see the many positive influences that the spirit of gratitude creates. In the hospitals and nursing homes throughout the world we see thousands upon thousands of health care workers and people in all professions touching lives and lifting spirits.

It is true that attitudes and practices of gratitude lead us on a soul-journey, in which we learn to live together as a people. I recall the play, *Hell is Other People*, written by philosopher and playwright Jean-Paul Sartre, and have always wondered how did he let his attitude perceive people from this negative side of the soul. My rebuttal to this would be "Hell is our Negative Attitude Toward Other People."

When we hold to the belief that all creation is holy in the sight of God, we, in the spirit of humility, express our gratitude to Him for making us a part (co-creators) of His creation. This is why ninety-nine percent of our prayers should be prayers of gratitude and praise.

Fortunately, caregiving experiences teach us this insight and wisdom through gratitude journal writing. The experiences indicate how sickness can spawn spiritual awakening, kindness, compassion, gratitude and humility. And writing about them, in quiet times, allows us the opportunity to see them for the excellent teachers they are.

3. "Let Thy Will Be Done"

Gratitude journal writing awakens us to fervently remember that two thousand years ago, our Savior Jesus Christ gave us the supreme lesson: "Let Thy will be done." Although millions of prayers have been offered to God, caregiving experiences teach us that no other prayer can be more fulfilling to the family caregiver than "Let Thy Will Be Done."

The spirit of gratitude opens our hearts to understand that there can be no better, no greater, no more fulfilling prayer than "Let Thy will be done."

An attitude of gratitude orders the caregiver's steps in the Word of God, teaching us by human experience that:

- When we love Eternal God, we become happy.

- When we love and serve Eternal God, we become happier.
- When we love, serve and surrender our individual will to Eternal God's Will, we become happiest.

We experience social and economic health when our attitude is gratitude in the workplace. When our profession is God's Will, we will feel a passion of inner joy or sense of satisfaction even before we begin doing it. This is an indication that the job is our spiritual mission, a divine gift from God. While working, we will also feel joy with a passion as we create, making our job a vocation in which we can touch the lives and lift the spirits of other people.

Finally, we will feel that we will be equally happy whether our service is fruitful or fruitless in the sight of man. We will feel independent of the favorable comments of others. Ordinarily, we' re happy only whenever humans praise us. But if we can have the same kind of passion and happiness, joy and satisfaction whether we succeed or fail in getting the praise of man, and if we can offer the results of our talents to Eternal God, then we will know that what we have done is His God's Will and that we are building for eternity by touching lives and lifting spirits.

4. Jesus of Nazareth, CEO

According to scripture, Jesus of Nazareth said to his disciples, "Follow me." And he as "president," took his twelve disciples and built one of the largest organizations the world has ever known, even most of us, especially us Christians, belong to Jesus' non-profit organization. In dynamic power and impact, we might think of it as a business.

When I say "one of the largest businesses the world has ever known," I mean no offense to Bill Gates, Microsoft CEO, and his comrades. But remember, it was Mr. Gates who showed us by example that his genius in modern technology is a direct line of creation from God through him to all mankind. We are grateful to Mr. Gates for using his miracle technology gift as a ministry for touching lives and lifting spirits. We are thankful to God for Mr. Gates and for giving him and other inventors and entrepreneurs like him the gift as an opportunity to touch lives and lift spirits.

Even Mother Teresa, CEO, whose ministry was a direct line of creation from God through her to us belongs to Jesus of Nazareth's worldwide non-profit organization. Mother Teresa took an oath of poverty, but she had control of millions of dollars that helped starving and ailing children. She, too, gave everyone an opportunity to use their abundant blessings to help the needy. Her "business" is still growing in abundance, and people from all walks of life are gladly contributing to this noble cause. She had a passion for her work to help to heal the world.

Even today we have *The Prayer of Jabez* author Bruce Wilkinson, CEO, an ordained Atlanta-based minister who teaches that God has unclaimed blessings waiting for all his children, has a massive non-profit organization. His ministry, which has become a direct line of creation from God through him to all mankind, extends an opportunity to everyone listening to help heal the self and the world.

Reverend Wilkinson's ministry extends to followers the opportunity to grow in faith and to use their abundant talents and gifts with a passion to help touch lives and lift spirits throughout the world in deeds of love and kindness. In his ministry, he focuses on two verses in the Old Testament that project the importance of having unshrinking faith in the goodness of God—1 Chronicles 4:9-10. Wilkerson uses these verses to write about the faith of Jabez, who was born in pain into the tribe of Judah. Rev. Wilkinson's message reiterates an attitude of gratitude that caregiving teaches: *pain and death are inevitable, but suffering is a choice because Jesus came that we might have life and have it abundantly.*

Jesus of Nazareth, CEO said, "Thy kingdom come, Thy will be done on earth as it is in heaven." Gratitude is the key that unlocks the gates (including Bill Gates) to heaven. Jesus also said that the kingdom of heaven is within us. *Blessed are your ears for they hear. —Matthew 13:16*

When we live with an attitude of gratitude and use our jobs as a ministry to help heal the world through acts of love and kindness, we can be assured that we are touching lives and lifting spirits, and we can be grateful because:

- We will be a blessing to God and to humanity.
- With an attitude of gratitude we will realize that all conditions of the world are within our control because we create our own reality.
- With an attitude of gratitude we will never be poor.
- With an attitude of gratitude we will always be humble before God, yet great in Him.
- With an attitude of gratitude we will awaken to an understanding that our job is a direct line of creation, from Eternal God through us to all mankind. We will always have critics, but so did Jesus. Being independent of the favorable comments of others, Jesus said, "Follow me." We are grateful that God has made us all co-creators of His creation and that He sent Jesus to teach us by example.
- With an attitude of gratitude we will awaken to a spiritual awareness that Our Eternal Father will see in us His aspiring creation, His transforming realization, His illumining revelation, His fulfilling manifestation and His candlelights for each new generation.

How well do I recall the childhood prayer that my younger sister Earline and I would often recite. It was her "Children's Day" speech and she had taught it to me.

God make my life a little light wherein the world to glow,
A tiny flame that burneth bright wherever I may go.
God make my life a little song that conquers all the sad,
That helps others to be strong and makes the singer glad.
God make my life a little flower that bringeth joy to all,
Content to bloom in natures bower
although its blooms be small.
God make my life a little prayer of tenderness and praise,
That teaches me to love and care
in all your wondrous ways.

Spiritual Key # 3

Kindness is the True Religion

Religion inspires man to live courageously and joyfully together on the face of the earth. — The Urantia Book.

Because your lovingkindness is better
than life, my lips shall praise thee.
—Psalm 63:3.

FOREWORD

Shared Wisdom from Family Caregiving

The world needs kindness. By being kind,
we have the power of making the world
a happier place in which to live.
—Father Lawrence G. Lovasik

Prelude

Troubled and confused by the world of violence, terrorism, wars and rumors of wars amid varying religious beliefs, the weary traveler asked, "Kind master, what can my disabled brother teach me about the world of religions and the various beliefs that are oftentimes overwhelmingly confusing?"

"My dear child," the Master answered, "as you care for your disabled brother, he will teach you that *universal kindness is the true religion.* But first, you must find your quiet space, be still and read about the various religions in order to increase your knowledge, wisdom and understanding about them. Then light your candle and begin writing your perceptions as you listen quietly to the spiritual meditations of your heart because within you are all the answers."

1. Kindness is our Spiritual Journey

In my world of family caregiving, I have found that one of the greatest gifts of caregiving experiences accompanied by gratitude journal writing is that it cultivates the powerful spirit of human kindness and gives one the bliss of divine life. Through these personal experiences, I have learned that God's love and kindness, often referred to as lovingkindness, is better than life.

Caregiving awakens us to the awareness that God wants to enter the world in us and through us; *He wants to be kind through us.* Why? Because, to the family caregiver, *kindness* is the power that wards-off caregiver-burnout and promotes inner peace.

In addition, kindness wins lost souls back to God by opening hearts that seemed empty, discouraged, disconnected, unloving, cold, frustrated and confused not only from caregiving, but from feeling emotionally bankrupt. We family caregivers who have experienced this awakening can share its wisdom with the world.

Jesus of Nazareth is the incarnate of kindness and has said to us, his suffering brothers, "follow me." We follow, but we seem to deliberately hide the power, purpose and spiritual importance of *kindness* which he so courageously taught us through his human examples. We need to capture his *kindness*, cultivate it, feel the love for it, and pass on its "candlelight of wisdom" to our younger generation, who will be our religious and political leaders of tomorrow.

Fortunately, family caregiving experiences have enabled us to awaken to the hidden power of kindness...kindness that can transform the world.

Kindness is spiritual. Studies show that most people want spirituality, but perhaps not in religious form. Many people leave church not because they have lost interest in spirituality, but because organized religion is not meeting their spiritual needs. In this twenty-first century, people are becoming more expressively spiritual. They, like John and me, are finding in spirituality what they are looking for in therapy—healing techniques and new inspiration.

It is for this reason I feel the spiritual need to write this chapter on kindness in which the world religions are presented to show their commonalities. By utilizing my personal format of gratitude journal writing, I find it easier to write deeply while meditating on wisdom gained from our world of family caregiver/patient experiences. On my spiritual journey, family caregiving has taught me that kindness is, indeed, the true religion, it is our spiritual journey.

Religion inspires us to live courageously and joyfully with each other on the face of the earth; it joins kindness with love, patience with compassion, insight with zeal, sympathy with power, and ideals with energy. It is impossible for us to wisely decide temporal issues or transcend the selfishness of personal interests unless we mediate prayerfully and ask for spiritual guidance.

PART ONE
Kindness Imparts True Wisdom

Behind the quest for spiritually lies a growing need for kindness, compassion and depth in our lives.

Prelude

And then the weary traveler asked, "Kind Master, in my family caregiving experiences, how can my disabled brother teach me the wisdom of kindness?"

The Master replied, "My child, your disabled brother will teach you that kindness is a virtue that embraces all virtues and is, therefore, the true religion. But in order to understand the spiritual messages of your caregiving experiences, you must continue to listen quietly, relax, meditate and pray as you begin your spiritual journey."

1. The Virtue of Kindness

Today, after staring into the flame of my candlelight and meditating for two hours, I feel the need to talk about kindness. Family caregiving has taught me through varying experiences that the virtue of kindness encompasses all virtues and is the true religion. Love is kind, thus, kindness is love in action. The Bible often speaks of God's lovingkindness.

Life has shown us that kindness has converted more souls to God than organized religions, zeal, eloquence, learning, adversity, pain, suffering or death.

Fortunately, I have learned that through gratitude journal writing, family caregiving experiences teach us by human examples that kindness stops the torrent of anger, frustrations, impatience, selfishness, ingratitude, racism, hate, prejudice, intolerance. Kindness drives gloom and darkness from souls and puts hope in fainting hearts. It lightens the burdens of weariness and depression and abates chronic depression and caregiver-burnout.

Family caregiving experiences show us by example the power of kindness and how it enables us to always *feel* the presence of God within that enables us to meet God in each other. It is our hope that this chapter will serve as a source of spiritual awakening to the reader, strengthening his insight that kindness is the true religion. Practicing kindness leads us to the heart of humanity and therefore to God.

2. By Being Unkind, What Have We Become?

As a family caregiver who, through gratitude journal writing, searches for the spiritual messages of our human experiences, I was deeply pained by the tragic news of five children who were drowned in a bathtub by their depressed mother. I was also painfully grieved to learn that their mother was a devoted family caregiver for her ailing father, who had just a month earlier died with Alzheimer's. She was, I am sure, a victim of postpartum depression and family caregiver-burnout.

Mainly, I decided to write this book to help awaken us all to what we have become because we have not cultivated the spirit of kindness; and to suggest what we, as the older generations, can do to help heal the world our young people are inheriting from us. The utter disregard for kindness is around us and, more than ever, includes the disrespect for life. Meanness is becoming the very fabric of our lives. The beast of meanness or unkindness is seen in schools, in magazines and movies and all over the world, even in the Holy Land where Jesus of Nazareth taught by example the power of human kindness. Why do we yet hide the power of kindness?

Is it any wonder that life, which God alone creates, has

now become disposable because of the messages we are sending to our younger generation?

Consider these unfortunate and heart piercing cases in which acts of unkindness prevailed where young mothers and young fathers destroyed human life with no regard to their own religious upbringing.

• A teenager and her boyfriend confessed to killing their baby in a motel and placing their baby in a dumpster, after the teenager asked her boyfriend to **"get rid of it."**

• A teenager had her baby during her high school prom, **tossed the baby in the restroom garbage**, and returned to boogie the night away.

• A teenager gave birth to a baby girl and asked her sister to **"bring me a knife so I can kill this thing."**

• A teenager **watched her baby drown in a toilet**.

• A teenager had her baby at the beach, brought him home in a duffel bag and **tossed him in the garbage**.

• A teenager didn't want to pay child support, so he **injected his 11-month-old son with the HIV virus**. His son is now doomed to a slow, tortuous death.

• A South Carolina mother **strapped her two sons in the back of her car** and pushed her car into a lake, drowning them both.

• A teenager who had an abortion at 16 and another at 17 said, **"I chose to deny them life, so that I could better my own."**

• A passenger at Boston's Logan Airport had her baby in the ladies room, **left her baby in the toilet** and boarded her flight to London.

• A teenager in Lake Worth gave birth to a baby boy, stuffed him in a garbage bag, and **tossed him over a six-foot fence**.

• A baby was **tossed down a trash chute** at a Key Biscayne, Florida, condo, causing the baby's death.

• A teenager gave birth, wrapped her baby boy in plastic bags, put him in a backpack **and threw him in a canal**. When the backpack would not sink, she went back home, placed a ten-pound weight in the backpack and tossed it in the canal. Her baby was discovered days later by an eleven-year-old who was fishing.

• In Fairfax, South Carolina, a baby was found clinging to life **buried in a shallow grave outside the trash dump**.

• A 15-year-old girl **stabbed her newborn baby to death** to keep a secret from her parents whom she feared and perceived as being very unkind.

• A 16-year old girl gave birth, then tossed her baby in a yard where a hungry pit bull **mauled her baby** beyond recognition.

It grieves our religious communities that our lack of human kindness has created a "culture of death" and has raised a generation of killers. What pains us even more is that this same young generation will be our leaders of tomorrow. Being raised with such an unkind attitude toward human life that they brought into the world, what do you think they, who will be our leaders of tomorrow in shaping the future of the world, will decide for us who have passed them the torch of religious and political leadership?

Our spiritual world is at risk. We need to stress that kindness to one another is, indeed, the true religion; and that kindness is love in action that leads us to the heart of humanity and, therefore, to God.

3. The Miracle of the Message

It was not a coincidence that I encountered a devout

parishioner at mass services the morning I was to begin writing this chapter with a passion for sharing knowledge on the power of human kindness. She was not aware that I was writing on the subject of kindness and humility of the soul when she handed me the August, 2001, edition of *The Christian Action News* with its philosophy of "Spreading the Word, Changing our World." I had been religiously meditating on the subject of kindness and humility, and had asked my Higher Source for divine guidance in helping me to share what caregiving experiences had taught me about the power of kindness and humility. Unfortunately, when I began my cross-section research to substantiate my findings, the library nor major bookstores had any appropriate literature on the subject of human kindness. The kind parishioner handed me the newsletter to read the article on stem cell research. But instead of reading that article, my eyes immediately caught articles entitled "The Hidden Power of Kindness," and a "Litany of Humility" that conveyed the identical messages that had been flooding my soul for months. With this miraculous and astounding answer to my prayer, I tearfully expressed my gratitude. Then through divine guidance, I began writing this book and completed it in three days. Later, I decided to include it in the Candlelights series.

As Descartes once said, *The thought will find itself a place*, especially when we are writing for Him in our mission to help spread the Word and change the world.

PART TWO
The Hidden Power of Human Kindness

As an elect of God, holy and beloved, put on tender mercies, kindness, humility, meekness, longsuffering, bearing with one another. (Colossians 3:12-13 NKJV).

Prelude

Feeling exhausted and confused by the various religions in his continuous search for God, the weary traveler asked, "Kind Master, why are there so many different religions in this world?"

The Master answered with *lovingkindness*, "They are here to teach you kindness, my child, so that you can be more *loving* to one another and a candlelight for the world. But first, you must be still, listen attentively and meditate prayerfully and silently, so that you will be awakened to transcendent wisdom, universal knowledge and most of all to spiritual understanding that undergirds *all* religions."

1. What is Kindness?

Kindness is God's love in action. It is the true, universal religion that unites us all as children of God. Kindness is the basic cause of God in the world.

Our Eternal Father wants to enter the world *in us and through us*; He wants to be *kind* through us.

In this week's issue of *The Florida Catholic*, the headline read: **Mideast violence: Past the point of no return?** In the article, the reporter stated that he heard a young man in his 20s, who was wearing a yarmulke, say he had just returned to the United States from living in Israel after several years. Surprisingly, the young man had served in the Israeli military and the reporter assumed he had duel citizenship. In talking with the gentleman about the Mideast crisis, the reporter perceived the vision of hope the young man was projecting in his courageous response. "Hopefully," he had sadly said to the reporter, "the situation would work itself out without too many people having to die."

This gentle response was enough to pierce the heart of any reader.

The reporter wrote "One thing is certain: For every new death we read about in the Holy Land, we can be sure that real peace becomes ever more elusive."

"But this is the Holy Land where Jesus of Nazareth taught us the power of kindness!" I said to my higher self, tears forming in my eyes. "Whatever happened to kindness?"

Yes, as children of the world, it is our mission to cultivate and express kindness in all our relationships with others. We can be as kind, merciful and gracious to others as Christ has been to us. Isn't this what the world of religion is all about?

According to the journalists, for every life taken in the Holy Land, there are significant consequences. Every religious body and nation should vigorously remind both sides—every Israeli and Palestinian—as well as all God's creation of religious faiths, of that simple fact.

If we are deeply concerned about the violence and suffering in the Mideast and throughout the world, we all need to closely adhere to the teachings of Jesus of Nazareth on his powerful message of kindness toward one another. While it is true that the old-time practices of silent prayer and withdrawal from the world are relevant in this twenty-first century; even more relevant is our kindness toward one another. To become fully human and achieve holiness, we must be present to our fellow man by meeting God in one another in the spirit of kindness. This is why *kindness* is the true religion.

2. *Kindness is...*

Kindness is, indeed, God's love in action. Fr. Lawrence G. Lovasik in his book, *The Hidden Power of Kindness*, tells us that kindness is the reason for God's presence in the universe; and that kindness is one of God's greatest gifts to humanity.

Kindness is the hidden power that enables us to meet God in one another. It is the most graceful attitude we can assume toward each other.

Yes, kindness is love in action. When we combine these two virtues, "love and kindness," we feel the overwhelming power of *lovingkindness* which is often spoken of in reference to God in the Holy Bible, especially in the Book of Psalms...Thy *lovingkindness*.

Kindness encompasses all the virtues of praise without its vices. Praise may encourage pride, but kindness enriches those who are kind to you. Kindness is the only kind of praise that is always and everywhere true. A kind word or deed, or even the mere tone of a kind voice is enough to convey sympathy to the suffering heart in its cry for help.

Kindness encompasses all religions without the dogma. Men may be charitable, merciful, compassionate, self-sacrificing, obedient to their religions' laws and orders, but yet not kind. Kindness stems from the depths of the heart where the spirit of our inner God dwells...the seat of the soul. Kindness is a grace always cultivated, even among people who are devout followers of God. Many devout people are unkind, even though they know that kindness is the ultimate cause of God in the world and in all religions.

As children of Eternal God, our mission in life should be to reconquer for His glory, through lovingkindness, his suffering, confused, and war-torn world. As a gift to Him, we should devote ourselves to the beautiful spirit of kindness so that all may enjoy the bliss of Divine life.

3. Kindness Wins Souls Back to God

Kindness is constantly winning more lost souls back to God by opening hearts and *feeling the love* within. Kindness is a love in action that touches lives and lifts spirits. Kindness has converted more lost souls to the spiritual life than organized religions, fame or fortune; sickness, suffering or death.

The downcast soul, when treated with kindness, is encouraged to be strong and to do bravely the very thing which, in an attitude of discouragement, it had almost resolved to leave undone. That spirit of encouragement may be the first link in the new chain that will lead him back to God, where love is always the only answer.

Fr. Lovasik tells us that the amount of kindness bears no proportion to the effect of kindness. It is not what we do, but how we do it that matters. The least kind action is greater than the greatest wrong. The smallest kindness can lift a heavy weight. It reaches far and travels swiftly. A kind action lasts a long period of time. The doing of it is only the beginning of a new world.

Kindness lifts the unfortunate, leads the wayward back to love and helps us to walk in the steps of Jesus of Nazareth, the incarnate of kindness, who taught us by example the power of kindness. Somehow, along the way, we humans seem to hide this very important power and its teachings.

The greatest work that kindness does to others is that it makes them kind themselves. The kindest people are those who have received the greatest number of kindnesses in their worlds. Kindness drives feelings of gloom, darkness, irritability disconnectedness, isolation, depression, detachment from troubled souls and restore them with hope.

With visions of hope, the troubled soul, after tasting the sweet fruit of kindness, returns to God and enters into His rest where inner peace abounds, and where loving God and obeying His will is a pleasure.

3. The Rewards of Kind Action

Family caregiving gives us many opportunities to cultivate the spirit of kindness; and to learn from daily experiences that kindness is one of God's most precious gifts to the world. We cannot pass a day without meeting opportunities for kind action. Everyday experiences of caregiving reveal that kind acts are as easy as they are frequent. Caregiving experiences reveal to us that when acts of kindness call for self-denial, the humbleness of sacrifice is noble and rewarding because kindness purifies, glorifies and ennobles all that it touches. Miraculously, we always gain inwardly and outwardly far more than what we lose. One act of kindness leads to another. A single act of kindness spreads its roots in all directions, and the roots spring up and make new trees. In essence, it lightens the burden of weariness that stems from caregivers' stress.

One of the greatest rewards of kindness is that it stops the growth of angry attitudes, takes the sting from failure, and kindles courageous ambitions to make one's life a blessing to humanity. It sweetens sorrow and lessens pain. It discovers unsuspected beauties of human character and calls forth the soul's highest response.

4. So, Whatever Happened to Kindness and Why is it Hidden?

Because Jesus Christ was kindness incarnate, and oftentimes we fail to follow him in our acts of kindness, we have lost the basic lesson he was trying to teach us by example. We seem to focus more on other aspects of his life, and fail to focus on his kindness and stress the importance of emulating this aspect of his character. Unfortunately, many of our religious leaders detest each other, yet they try to teach us followers how to love one another. That kind of negative energy flowing from our religious leaders only drives the would-be followers away from God. It gets all in the ceilings, walls, lights and everything it touches.

In addition and sadly enough, we have followers of many religious faiths who think their faith is superior to their neighbors' religious faiths. They are afraid to "kill with kindness and humility" the ego-thief within. They haven't awakened to the awareness that all creation is holy. This level of awakening is the result of deep and continuous spiritual meditation with a heart of humility.

Kindness is Christ's basic law and is a sign of greatness. We must always remember that kindness is love in action toward others, and that it is in kindness toward one another that we meet God.

Throughout the Old Testament the words "steadfast love," "mercy," and "kindness" are used interchangeably. The prophets tell us that kindness is the persistent effort of God to reach His people and enable them to return to Him.

Jesus of Nazareth came to earth to express kindness. He lived to model it. He died to offer it. And he has returned to impart it to us in the Holy Spirit.

Let us examine the life of Paul. His bitter, iron-clad, negative attitude toward others and himself had been melted by an overwhelming act of kindness by Jesus who met him on the road to Damascus and converted him. Afterwards, Paul became one of the kindest and greatest prophets in the history of Christianity. He wrote the Epistles (sermons/letters) to the Corinthians, Ephesians, Philippians, Colossians, Thessalonians; to Timothy, The Hebrews, Titus, Philemon.

His letters are some of the greatest books in the Holy Bible.

Our Heavenly Father never demands anything of us that He is not willing to give us. Kindness is a gift he gave us. It is implanted, ingrained and imputed into our divine heredity. Kindness is our true nature; it is our inheritance. It is ours to cultivate and share in all our relationships with others. If we pray and meditate daily, we can be as kind, loving and merciful as God is to us because He will help us.

Jesus has shown us the way to *feel* the kindness within us; and that kindness is a sign of greatness. Therefore, let us take the labels off our minds and step boldly into our greatness that stems from spiritual deeds of kindness.

Let us always remember that when Jesus came into the world, there were few institutions of mercy, hospitals or mental institutions, or places of refuge for the poor. There were few homes for the orphans and few havens for the forsaken and disabled. In his day, it was a cruel, heartless world that showed no kindness or compassion for the less fortunate. Jesus changed that by showing us by example the power of his kindness and love...lovingkindness. His ministry was a direct line of creation, from God through him to a suffering humanity.

And now, wherever true Christianity has gone, Jesus' followers have performed acts of kindness and gentleness to others throughout the world.

"Follow me." Jesus said. Let us follow him anew, embracing the spiritual power of his kindness... the pathway to finding God within ourselves in lovingkindness to our fellow man.

PART THREE

Kindness Encompasses All Virtues and Religions

The greatest work that kindness does to others is that it makes them kind themselves. Kindness is one of God's greatest gifts to the world. —Fr. Lawrence G. Lovasik

Prelude

And then the weary traveler asked, "Kind Master, how do the various religions of the world teach us kindness when they all have so many different paths that lead to you?"

In the spirit of lovingkindness, the master softly whispered, "My child, your brother, Jesus, who is the incarnation of God, said to you, 'In my Father's house are many mansions; if it were not so, I would have told you.' Quietly listen to him and prayerfully meditate on the world's religions. But first, you must be humble, and in your state of humility, your thirst for spiritual understanding will be quenched by various teachers who will appear."

1. Kindness and the World's Religions

Seek for yourself, O man; search for your own true self.
He who seeks shall find—but marvel and joy, he will not find himself he will find God, or, if he finds himself, he will find himself in God.
—St. Augustine

Saturday, August 11, 2001

When, through gratitude journaling, the experiences of family caregiving led me to feel the need for a higher level of understanding of myself and the daily lessons that religion is teaching us on our journey, I was mesmerized by a phrase that came to me: *Kindness is the true religion.* Kindness is an attitude that enables us to respect, love and appreciate others and their religions. It is a quality of behavior that stands firm without forcing others to their knees. Kindness is the spirit of love at work within all religions.

Love is a universal language in which the power of human kindness is hidden. All the religions of the world believe in kindness because it is our divine inheritance. Whether or not it is practiced and to what extent is an individual choice.

As chairperson of Ecumenism and Evangelism for the Miami Archdiocesan of Catholic Women, I had the opportunity to study the various religions and found that they all teach the virtue of kindness toward one another. Whether or not it is religiously practiced every day in our relationships with others is another story. In reading about the various religions, I was led to understand why people have different views about the Universe and its source, which many of us call God. At the heart of all religions is the belief in something bigger than us who takes care of all of us...a Universal Caregiver.

Unfortunately, religious enthusiasm has caused the death of millions of people who have fought on the side of one religion, or faith system, against another. It is our hope that in this twenty-first century, most faiths will encourage their members to try to understand, respect and appreciate other people's beliefs and treat each other with kindness. Many people see their spiritual journey as a search to learn to love unconditionally, to be kind and compassionate toward others and to forgive. They all believe in the universal wisdom of treating others as they wish to be treated. We need to feel the love within—that love is the light with which we light our candles so that they can shine into the world of darkness.

We all want to be treated with love and kindness. Kindness is a state of being unruffled and unflappable. In many messages in the Scriptures, it is linked with love as in *lovingkindness*.

Kindness is behavior that flows from agape, God's love. It is behavior that is holy, pure, gentle and basically rooted in good and for the good of another person. While it is true that love might cause one to make difficult decisions or exercise behavior that might be perceived as harsh, "kindness" refers to loving behavior that is compassionate, gentle and loving.

2. Faith Systems and the Spirit of Kindness

In my caregiving experiences and gratitude journal writing, I have been joyfully awakened to the belief that Jesus Christ of Nazareth is the incarnation of God and of kindness. Because of his teachings of kindness, he has the largest number of followers in the world (over 840 million) compared to other faith systems. Christianity has its roots in Judaism because Jesus' ancestors were Jews, and Jesus himself was a Jew. Christianity centers on the belief that Jesus Christ is the Son of God. I have been taught to believe that all the generations of the world are descendants of the Prophet Abraham.

The various faith systems of the world include Christianity, Judaism; Baha'i, Buddhism, Confucianism, Cynicism, Hinduism, Islam, Kabbalah, Shintoism, Sikhism, Shinto, Suduanism (Jainism) Taoism, Voudouism, and Zoroastrianism.

There are others such as Maori, Australian Spirituality, Native American Beliefs, The New Age, Kwanzaa, and Scientology that are said to be more a philosophy of life rather than a religion.

And because my faith is Christianity with its roots in Judaism, I feel the need to share an outline of the two faiths and their interconnectedness. Afterwards, I will share a brief statement about some of the other faiths thus mentioned to show our human interconnectedness, interrelatedness and interdependence in relation to their teachings of kindness.

CHRISTIANITY

Christians beliefs are founded on the teachings of Jesus Christ as set forth in the New Testament. Christianity teachings are also based on the Hebrew Bible or Old Testament. Its doctrines teach God's love for humanity and stress the importance of kindness and brotherly love. Christians believe in social justice, universal peace and brotherly love.

Today, Christianity has about 300 denominations. "In my Father's house there are many mansions..."

1. God Concept - Monotheistic (one God)
   a. This one God is in 3 persons (personalities) which are most predominant: God as Creator—(Father, Redeemer (son), Sanctifier (spirit) - Trinitarian. Jesus came to earth as the incarnation of God. He taught by human examples the virtues of love, kindness, humility, truth, forgiveness and all of God's treasury of virtues.

2. Cosmos - Created by God
   a. Some fundamentalists take the creation story literally - Literalist
   b. Contextualist - text and context, (i.e., Catholics - day + symbol)

3. Humanity - Created in the image and likeness of God
   a. Superior to creation (we humans have a soul, we are higher beings).

4. Plight is Sin
   a. Salvation from this plight comes from Jesus, who freed us from our sinfulness and taught us how to love God and one another.
   b. Code of Conduct - In order to accept your salvation, you must try to follow The Way. (Jesus, The Way, taught us to love God and our neighbor).
   C. Destiny - resurrection of the body.
   D. Sacred Book - The Holy Bible - helps us to know our story and the story of God in our life.

JUDAISM

Judaism was one of the first religions to emphasize ethical monotheism, or the belief in One God who is just, kind and good. It was the first religion to speak of God's lovingkindness. The Jewish religion centers around this belief.

1. God Concept - Monotheistic (Fear God and keep His commandments, for this is the whole duty of man. Love your neighbor as yourself).
   a. This God is a personal God.

2. Cosmos - created by God, "It is good."

3. Humanity - created in the image and likeness of God.
   a. Humanity is the ruler of the cosmos.

4. Plight is sin
   a. Salvation means being freed from all sinfulness.
   b. code of Conduct - observing the Law.
   c. Destiny - union with God.
   d. Sacred Book - Torah - tells how God intervened in the past and how we must act today because of the law. The Torah contains a code of conduct for

humankind, emphasizing the importance of being kind to one another.

5. Kabbalah - A medieval philosophy that has transcended Jewish interest.

Thousands of Jewish people left organized religion in the 1960s and 1970s because they felt there was something spiritually lacking. Many of them felt that organized religion was not giving then the spiritual tools to make their worlds more adaptable to modern life. But within the last ten years, Jewish mysticism, known as Kabbalah, has drawn many back into the fold. Kabbalah, an increasingly popular Jewish mystical tradition that developed in the thirteenth century, offers a spiritual basis for all Jewish practices and traditions. Followers feel that there is no real understanding of why one is Jewish without it. The new popularity of Kabbalah among Jews and non-Jews like Median who is Catholic, shows that people are searching for deeper meanings. More than twenty-nine new Kabbalah meeting places have opened in the last year around the country.

BAHA'I

Founded by Baha'u'llah, the Baha'i Faith is the newest of world religions, and stresses the oneness of all mankind. Only recently has the public come to recognize that it is, in fact, a major religion—one worthy of study and reflection.

Baha'u'llah called all people to give up their prejudices and to recognize the fellowship of all humankind as children of one loving God. He said the time has come for humanity to unite under one common faith. He revealed a plan for world civilization to be built on a foundation of love, kindness and justice.

Among the most fundamental of Baha'u'llah's teachings are these:

- There is only one God.
- All religions share a common foundation.
- Humanity is one. People of all races, nations, economic groups, and religious backgrounds are equal in the sight of God.

And:

- Each individual is responsible for investigating truth independently.
- Science and religion are in harmony. Science without religion is materialism — religion without science is superstition.
- Women and men are equal, like the two wings of one bird.
- Every child is entitled to a sound, basic education.
- There is a spiritual solution to economic problems.
- The world needs an international auxiliary language.
- We must establish a universal peace protected by a world commonwealth.

People of all backgrounds, as Baha'is, are striving to develop the potential to rise above the division and prejudice of the world to become lovers of all humankind.

BUDDHISM

In Buddhism, wakefulness is the way of life. Buddhists believe in truth and a way of life, rather than a God or gods. They believe that the root of all problems in life is suffering which is caused by materialism—the desire to own objects. To eliminate suffering caused by materialism, Buddhists follow eight laws known as the Eightfold Path. These laws are as follows:

1. Right Understanding
2. Right Thought
3. Right Speech
4. Right Action
5. Right Livelihood
6. Right Effort
7. Right Mindfulness
8. Right Concentration

Buddhists believe in the power of meditating on justice and mercy; and that faith is man's true wealth because it is the endowment of virtue and glory. Two of their favorite quotes that highlight kindness to others are: " Do not to others those things you would not want done to you." "See yourself in others; who then can you harm?"

CONFUCIANISM

This faith is based on the belief and teaching of Confucius, a Chinese sage who believed that the young should respect their elders and ancestors, and that we should behave toward others as we would like them to behave toward us. Some scholars consider Confucianism a system of ethics rather than a religion, because Confucius taught more about how men should act toward one another than about God. Confucius believed in a Supreme Being to which he prayed.

HINDUISM

Hinduism, the traditional religion of India, is one of the oldest religions in the world. Its teachings are found in a book called Bhagavad-Gita, which tells of a conversation between a person and God.

Hindus believe we have many different lives, so that we can learn spiritual lessons through our human experiences on earth. The Great Controller is the generator of all things—all evolves from Him. And this is the sum of duty: "Let no man do to another what would be repugnant to himself; cherish no malice, smite not him who smites you, conquer anger with mercy, and vanquish hate by benevolence. All this we should do because God is a kind friend and a gracious father who remits all our earthly offenses."

Hinduism centers on belief on the sacredness of all living things.

ISLAM

The Muslim religion is based on human beings having a connection with Allah, the Arabic name for God. The prophet Mohammed was chosen by Allah to lead the Islamic faith, and his teaching is very popular in the Arab world. Prior to this, Mohammed was a successful businessman. History tells us that during a pilgrimage, the Archangel Jibriel, also known as Gabriel, visited Mohammed and gave him divine messages. The Koran, the book in which Muslim teachings are recorded, is highly treasured because its teaching is said to reveal the character of God. They believe in serving God and obeying His commandment to love one another through acts of human kindness. Followers of Islam believe in meditation, prayer and fasting

JAINISM

Like Buddhism, Jainism is a code for living rather than a religion. Jains say that we are all divine and we can get in touch with our spiritual side by releasing the soul. The Great Vows that Jains take include telling the truth, avoiding violence, not taking anything unless it is given, and being detached from people, places and things. They embrace the theory that "Nothing belongs to us, except in memory."

SHINTOISM

Shintoism is the traditional faith of the Japanese people and is based on the elements of Nature. Shintoists believe that there is healing power in the mountains, streams, wind and trees; and that there are four kinds of worship: cleansing, offering, prayer and feasting.

Shinto means "The Way of God." Shinto teaches loyalty to beloved places and traditional Japanese ways of life. Shintoists worship many gods, including emperors, national heroes of the past and various nature deities.

SIKHISM

Sikhism is a religion in Northwest India and is a blend of Hinduism and Islam, believing in one God and the transmigration of the soul. A Sikh believes that all people are equal in the eyes of God. Sikhs, Hindus and Buddhists believe that every soul has more than one Earthly life, and is reborn after death. The first leader was Guru Nanak who taught people to find happiness through repeating the name of God.

TAOISM

The balance between Yin and Yang—the negative and positive forces of creation—is at the heart of Chinese Taoism. A Taoist seeks to feel peaceful and calm on the inside, whatever is going on in his or her life. Taoists are taught how everything in the world is connected by reading *The I Ching*, or *Book of Changes*.

VOUDOUISM

Voudouism is the name given to a set of religious beliefs and the practice of magic of certain African tribes; and is most popular in Haiti. The word is a West African word which means *god* or *spirit*. Millions of followers around the world believe that the work of the gods appears in every part of life. Voudounists believe that a Supreme Being, called Gran Met, made the world, and that the spirits of the dead live in a world of spirits but can visit the world of the living to extend help.

ZOROASTRIANISM

The followers of the prophet called Zoroaster, or Zarathustra, are known as Zoroastrians. In the tenth century, Zoroastrians, called Parsees, fled from prosecution by Muslims from Persia to India. They believe the most important thing in life is to take responsibility for our actions.

This religion centers around the god of right-consciousness and light. Zoroastrianism teaches that people can attain eternal reward in heaven by supporting the god of right-consciousness and light in his battle against the powers of evil. Zoroastrianism doctrines of heaven, hell and the devil had some influence on Christianity.

2
Additional Systems of Beliefs and Customs

AUSTRALIAN SPIRITUALITY

Aboriginal Australians communicate with their gods through art and dance. They believe strongly in dreams, prayers, brotherhood, and rituals; and that the ancient paths still sing a song about the creation of the land. They meditate in solitude for long periods of time to help them connect with the universe and its source.

KWANZAA

This African-American cultural celebration is based on seven laws which teach the art of living in the community with family and friends, creatively working, and faith in God.

The Principles of Kwanzaa are:

1. Unity —To strive for and maintain unity in the family, community, nation and race.
2. Self-Determination — to define ourselves, name ourselves, create for ourselves, and speak for ourselves.
3. Collective Work and Responsibility — To build and maintain our community together and to make our brothers' and sisters' problems our problems, and to solve them together.
4. Cooperative Economics — To build and maintain our own stores, shops and other businesses, and to profit together from them.
5. Purpose — To make as our collective vocation the building and developing of our community in order to restore our people to their traditional greatness.
6. Creativity — To do always as much as we can, in the way that we can, in order to leave our community more beautiful and beneficial than when we inherited it.
7. Faith — To believe with all our hearts in our parents, our teachers, our leaders, our people, and the righteousness and victory of our struggle.

In the traditional religions of Africa, God is seen as the mother and father of the universe. It is traditional Africans' belief that God is in everything and that everything is in God. Therefore, they have a high interest in nature. The ancestors are known to be guardians of the spirit and pass on to everyone the energy of the Divine.

MAORI

In New Zealand, the Maori people believe in legends

and myths. They believe that Mother Earth and Father Sky are the creator gods and were separated by their sons, who in turn created the human race. They believe that all creation is a gift from the gods, and that followers should obey the moral laws of the gods and the tribe. Maori people sometimes wear a Heitiki around their necks that represents a human embryo, or a still-born child. They believe the spirit of still-born children to be very powerful and pure because they were cheated of life on earth.

NATIVE AMERICAN BELIEFS

For the Native Americans who live among nature and spend much of their time in silence, everything in life is sacred. Native Americans have a strong connection to the elements and to the animal world. In their world, they believe that life is a spiritual journey which involves one's mind, body, and spirit. They call this belief an Earth Walk. The spiritual activities of the Native Americans include using tools such as herbs, sacred pipes, and feathers. In their native world, they perform powerful chants and creative dances.

Below are the Ten Commandments of Native Americans. This code of ethics embodies the basic principles of kindness.

The Ten Native American Commandments

These Ten Commandments from Native American cultures contain such profound truths they can be found on posters and inscribed on various objects throughout the world.

- TREAT the earth and all that dwell thereon with respect.
- REMAIN close to the Great Spirit.
- SHOW great respect for your fellow beings.

- WORK together for the benefit of all mankind.
- GIVE assistance and kindness wherever needed.
- DO what you know to be right.
- LOOK after the well-being of mind and body.
- DEDICATE a share of our efforts to the greater good.
- BE truthful and honest at all times.
- TAKE full responsibility for your actions.

THE NEW AGE OF THE 21st CENTURY

According to "New Age" believers, we humans are all connected to the same source, and we should try to look to the universe mystically, rather than scientifically. People of the New Age take a holistic approach to life. In their new age world they try to achieve global consciousness, or an awareness of the universe and everything that lives in it.

Religions/Kindness

Thus, we can see that practically all religions reflect a philosophy of kindness and try to instill this spiritual message in their followers. They reflect the type of kindness that pervades and penetrates the whole nature. Kindness washes away all the negative feelings and attitudes and replaces them with love, humility, understanding and compassion. We treat others as we wish to be treated when we practice kindness.

When we reflect on our life which is given by God to spread love, we know the necessity of being a vessel into which God can pour his spirit of kindness; and we are commanded to use his spirit of kindness in our relationships with others. We know that we receive our fullest relationship with God by constantly practicing an attitude of kindness toward each other. Human kindness is possible only in an attitude of thoughtfulness that is sensitive to the unique nature of others.

The virtue of kindness toward one another is written in most of our religious doctrines.

Whenever we recognize that the dominant feeling in our heart is often a feeling of contempt, dislike or cruelty, we should ask ourselves, "Do I *feel* the feeling of kindness within, or do I *feel* a feeling of unkindness, contempt, dislike or just plain cruelty?" The heart always speaks the truth. This is why meditation is so important. It gives us the opportunity to sit still and listen to our true inner feelings.

The more we look into our own lives, the more we become aware of how often and how many people we have inwardly rejected. Oftentimes this dreadful feeling of our own cold-cold hearts can increase to the point that we ask ourselves, "Why do I *feel* so unkind today?" "Why am I such that I offend or hurt my best friend?" "Why do I *feel* like an empty shell inside?" What a blessing to realize that we create our own happiness by changing our perceptions. Knowing that feelings of kindness make us happy, we can tell our hearts to *feel* the inherited kindness that God has already given us as a precious gift.

Yes, we have the gift of *feeling* the spirit of kindness within us. We have to nourish it daily because it contains our joy, happiness, peace, abundant life, and all the promises of God.

Oftentimes we wonder about the reported evil in the world that floods the news media, especially the Middle East violence in the so-called Holy Land among *devout religious groups*. We ask, "If God is all-kind, all-loving and all-powerful, how can He allow religious men to be so evil to one another...especially religious brothers who are spiritual leaders?" The answer is: we have to read the spiritual message through meditation and prayers as we work with the leaders in every way possible to establish peace. We are our brother's keeper, and with the help of each other, we are evolving. We are God's kingdom. *Thy kingdom come; Thy will be done on earth as it is in heaven.*

We must continue to evolve religiously, following in the footsteps of courageous leaders who have fought the good fight with deeds of love and mercy, kindness and humility. Yes, we are evolving; and in the words of Ernest W. Shurtleff who wrote the song, *Lead On, O King Eternal,* we humbly say...

For not with swords' loud clashing, nor roll of
stirring drums, But deeds of love and mercy,
Thy heavenly kingdom comes.

PART FOUR
Kindness and the Unity of Religions

The power of kindness is not in what it does for us, but where it leads us; at once to the heart of humanity and therefore to God.

Prelude

And then the weary traveler asked, "Kind Master, how are these various religions unified in their mission to teach us kindness toward one another?"

The kind Master replied, "My child, listen pensively to their messages and meditate on them that you might understand why they all embrace the spirituality of kindness."

1. Awakening to the Spirituality of Kindness

Today, I feel the need to light my candle and mediate deeply on the lessons I have learned about the various religious beliefs and practices. Family caregiving experiences have awakened me to a need to further understand all aspects of religion and the unification of religions so that I can share my findings with others, especially other family caregivers. Inasmuch as we are candles in search for light that gives us all inner peace, we know that the light comes from within. It shines even brighter when we understand the kindness and unity of religions, and that kindness, although hidden, is the spiritual basis of all religions.

In my world of caregiving, journal writing is often a form of deep meditation based on cross-section research. The following pattern will attest to this procedure.

2. Religious Beliefs and Practices

Religion and the Individual. Almost all religions place great emphasis on the individual. All religions try to offer their followers a set of values by which to live. They emphasize ethical conduct and give the individual a framework for judging right from wrong and for living a good life. Through their emphasis on the Supreme Being, they give the individual reasons for living a good life and for treating others as they themselves wish to be treated.

As earlier implied, man will meet God only through his neighbor, for there he will find Christ. His fully human life on earth is the most perfect example for all humanity and the ideal on which man must model his own life in order to realize complete growth as a human being and attain that true holiness which the person of Christ epitomizes.

The Deity. While it is true that, sooner or later, most humans come to believe that their lives depend on forces in the world more powerful than themselves they identify these powers with reverence and seek good relations with them by being obedient.

These forces then become their gods. People who do not believe that there is a God are known as atheists. Atheists believe in love, but they do not accept the belief that God is love. Others, called agnostics, do not deny God, but say that it is impossible for man to know whether there is a God and a spiritual world. Sometimes, like many who have chosen to believe in God, they might embrace the hypothesis: "The only truth we know is that we do not know."

Many primitive people believe that a vague, general, powerful living but impersonal force exists in the world. On a higher level, some people accept a belief in many gods. They worship the basic powers of nature.

Most major religions today reject the idea of many gods. They accept monotheism and say that all the world's powers are expressions of a single, Supreme Being. Christianity,

Judaism, Islam, Baha'i and Zoroastrianism believe that God is all-good and all-powerful, and rules the world with a conscious purpose. They perceive Him as pure spirit and no body at all. Such religions as Taoism, Buddhism, Hinduism and some forms of Confucianism teach that personality traits of any sort suggest man rather than God. Followers of Confucianism believe that Confucius' teachings lead to perfection in man's relationship with other men.

Codes of Conduct. Every religion teaches its followers how they should behave. Some religious codes tell people how to act toward God. The various religions differ on many points as to what their followers should or should not do. Most of them speak of man's relationship with man with emphasis on kindness, especially those religions that believe in the oneness of God.

The Oneness of God. Organized religion depends on education for its existence. Each generation must teach its religion to the next generation. Religions that believe in the oneness of God stress this belief in their basic religious text—the Secret Book—that is handed down from generation to generation. These religions teach the lovingkindness of God and the importance of meeting God in man through acts of kindness.

- "The Lord our God is one Lord." (Christ, New Testament, Mark 12:29)
- "But, just how many Gods are there...?" "One" (Hinduism, Brihan-Aranyaka Upanishad 3:9:1)

- He is God, the One and Only; God the Eternal, Absolute...and there is none like unto Him." (Muhammad, 570-632 A.D., Koran 112:1-4)

- No God is there beside Thee, the Supreme Ruler, the All-Glorious, the Omniscient." (Bah'u'llah, Prayers and Mediations, p. 6)

- "I am the Lord, and there is none else, there is no God beside me." (Judaism, Isaiah 45:5)

- There is O monks, an Unborn, Unoriginated, Uncreated, Unformed." (The Buddha, c. 560-480 B.C., Udana 80-81)

3. Kindness and the Oneness of Humanity

In early religions, men were concerned with only the other persons in their groups. Later, religions taught love, kindness and service to all humanity. A world-wide stress on ethical teaching occurred between 1000 and 500 B.C., with the Hebrew prophets preaching in Palestine and Zoroastrianism developing in Persia, Buddhism and Jainism in India, and Confucianism in China. Jesus of Nazareth taught us by human examples the wisdom of kindness and service to all humanity during his short stay here on earth.

Many religions teach the oneness of humanity and the importance of treating others with kindness just as we wish to be treated. They emphasize that we meet God in each other through acts of kindness; and that kindness is love in action. These codes of conduct are passed down from generation to generation and is repeatedly stated in the Sacred Book of each religion. The following are examples:

- Be united in your purpose, let your hearts be as one heart, minds of all as one mind, so that your affairs may be cooperatively well organized." (Hinduism, Krishna, Rig Veda 8:7)

- "Ye are the fruits of one tree, and the leaves of one branch...the earth is but one country, and mankind is its citizens." (Baha'u'llah, 1617-92, gleanings from the Writings of Baha'u'llah, pp. 218, 250).

- "Have we not all one father? Hath not one God created us? Why do we deal treacherously every man against his brother...? (Judaism, Malachi 2:10).

- " God...hath made of one blood all nations of men for to dwell on all the face of the earth." (Paul, New Testament, Acts 17:26).

- "Ye are all parts one of another." (Muhammad, Koran 3:195).

- "Do not be angry, nor should ye secret resentment bear, for as a mother risks her life and watches over her child, so boundless be your love to all, so tender, kind and mild." (The Buddha, Suttanipata, V. 148).

PART FIVE

Kindness: Humility of Heart

True humility is the feeling of oneness.
Humility means giving kindness and joy to others.

Prelude

And the weary traveler, thirsting for more enlightenment, then asked, "Kind master, with so many religions that teach us kindness, please tell me what is the real secret of the spiritual life of kindness?"

The kind master smiled, then softly replied, "Humility, my dear child, is the real secret of the spiritual life of kindness. But you must be still, pray and meditate silently to feel the spirit of humility in the depths of your heart, and let it transform you."

1. Kindness and the Virtue of Humility

Sri Chinmoy, in his book, The *Wings of Joy*, tells us that humility is the jewel of kindness and is, indeed, the real secret of the spiritual life. The ego talks, but humility acts from the inner world of kindness.

When we embrace the spirit of humility, we neither underestimate nor overestimate our life. Humility is not a matter of being weak or wimpish, it is our feeling of consecrated oneness with humanity.

Humility with acts of kindness is the spirit of God that dwells within us. It is a gift of love. Sri Chinmoy tells us that "Real humility is the expansion of our consciousness," and that the higher we go, the greater is our promise to the Supreme in mankind.

Life teaches us that the more light we receive by virtue of our humility and kindness, the more we have to offer humanity.

2. Humility of Kindness is the Soul's Strength

Soulful humility is a form of divine power. Many prophets and gurus possess it. Jesus of Nazareth has shown us that what we call "humility" in heaven, we call "strength" on earth. Jesus of Nazareth has also shown us that when the soul's strength manifests, it does so through the spirit of humility. Humility means oneness with the rest of the world. On the strength of our kindness and humility we are tremendously enlarged. "He that humbles himself shall be exalted."

A prophet or guru is someone who is kind, humble and important in a religion, faith or philosophy. Prophets are known to be humble, kind and wise individuals who speak through divine inspiration or receive messages from a Higher Source.

Prophets usually have many followers and belong to a religion. Gurus give spiritual guidance to a smaller number of believers and may not be linked with a religion other than one which they themselves founded.

SECTION 2
The Kindness and Humility of Prophets and Gurus

"...and he that shall humble himself shall be exalted."
— Matthew 23:12b

1. Faith Founders

The following are brief statements of various faith founders who exerted the spirit of kindness and humility. Their lives are examples of strength, greatness and wisdom that grew out of acts of kindness and humility of spirit. Their humble and profound leadership still teaches us that their ministry was always a direct line of creation from God through them to humanity.

• ***The Prophet Abraham*** was the ancestor of the Israelite people. His name was originally Abram, signifying *high father.* The book of Genesis states that God later changed it to Abraham which means "father of many nations." After the death of his father, he moved to Palestine, obeying a command of God. There, he built his first altar at the town of Bethel. Abraham's courageous life is told in Genesis which shows him as the representative man of faith. He ranks among the greatest men in Hebrew history.

• ***Moses***, the great leader and prophet, helped the Jewish people to escape from Egyptian slavery. God gave Moses The Ten Commandments on Mount Sinai and he recorded them on tablets of stone. The Ten Commandments is a body of moral and religious laws set forth in the Old Testament. These laws governed the ancient Israelites and later became the basic principles of Judaism and Christianity.

• ***Jesus Christ*** founded the Christian faith. In clearer terms, Christianity is the religion founded by the apostle Paul upon the teachings of Jesus Christ. Jesus began his ministry in Palestine, instructing and preaching to people about the Kingdom of God. He traveled around the country with a group of twelve chosen followers called disciples whom he anointed to preach his doctrine. In line with the teachings of the Old Testament prophets, Jesus insisted upon justice toward men and humanity, and toward God. He taught by human examples the love of God for all people of the world. He and his disciples traveled around the world giving kind and humble services, preaching and teaching by examples the Word of God and His lovingkindness; healing and performing miracles, showing compassion with acts of love and concern for the sick and disabled.

The Jewish leaders of Jesus' time did not approve of his claim that he was the Messiah, the promised deliverer of the Jews. Roman authorities feared that because of his divine power and huge number of dedicated followers, he meant to lead an uprising against Roman rule in Palestine. Therefore, he was tried, condemned to death and crucified. Christianity spread rapidly, due to the work of Saint Paul and other apostles. Christianity is the most widespread religion in the world and has influenced government, thought and art for almost 2,000 years. The three great divisions of Christianity today are the Roman Catholic Church, the Eastern Orthodox Church and the Protestant denominations.

• ***The Dalai Lama*** (Dalai means "ocean of wisdom") is the supreme leader for Tibetan Buddhists and a living example of wisdom and kindness for others to follow. His position is earned in childhood through remembering past incarnations; and his wisdom, kindness and humility inspire people from all over the world and across all cultures. At a very young age, a potential Dalai can recall objects, places and people he knew in a past life. Today, the present Dalai Lama is the monk called Tenzin Gyatso. Born in 1935, the Dalai Lama has been living in exile in the Himalayas since the Chinese invasion of Tibet. In 1989, he was awarded the prestigious Nobel Peace Prize.

• ***Mohammed*** was the Prophet of Islam and the founder of the Islam, a religion based on the idea of the unity of God and the brotherhood of man. Born in southwestern Arabia, Mohammed was repelled by idol worship and spent hours in religious meditation. A kind and humble servant, he received messages from an angel while sitting in a cave in Mount Hirae. He became convinced that there is only one God and that He had revealed himself in the Bible. He was told to tell the people that there is only one God, who became known to those who followed His teachings as Allah. Mohammed preached the Ten Commandments of the Old Testament. He abolished the customs of worshiping idols and killing girls at birth. He limited the practice of polygamy, or marriage to two or more wives, and restricted divorce. He reformed inheritance laws, regulated slavery, gave help to the poor and the oppressed. He approved war and conquest in the case of self-defense, but allowed Jews and Christians to practice their beliefs and keep their property if they surrendered. Practitioners of the religion he founded are known as Muslims.

• ***Guru Nanak*** was the first teacher of Sikhism. He believed that all people are united in God's eyes, and he gave this message to the Hindus and Muslims who lived in what is now known as Pakistan. Because of his kindness, humility and wisdom, nine more Sikh gurus have followed him.

• ***Siddhartha Gautama***, later known as Buddha, was an Indian prince brought up in great wealth. In his spirit of kindness and humility, he saw the suffering of his people. He gave up his riches and went on a journey around India, and eventually founded Buddhism, a philosophy based on "The truth."

• ***Jacob*** was the son of Isaac and grandson of the prophet Abraham. He was later given the name *Israel* by God, and the people of Israel named their nation after him.

• ***Mother Meer***, sometimes known as "The Divine Mother," is revered by followers of all professions across the globe. By many followers, she is believed to be a supreme being who has come to live on earth to help suffering people in search for their higher selves. It is said that Mother Meer has a miraculous healing light which she uses to help the earth and its people. It is her firm belief that our connectedness with God or the Divine is most important for our spiritual growth, and especially for our transformation and awakening, or for unlocking our divine inheritance to abundant life as we courageously rise to our highest potentials.

• ***Sai Baba*** is known as a supreme being who was incarnated in the world to help people rediscover the wisdom of ancient Hindu teachings. He believes that we are all part of God, and we should recognize this and learn to love one another.

• ***Charles Taze Russell*** is the founder of the Jehovah's Witnesses movement. He believes strongly that people should prepare themselves spiritually for the apocalypse, the end of the world. The religion teaches the lovingkindness of Jehovah, a life of spiritual discipline, and the brotherhood of man.

• ***Rajneesh*** — Bhagwam Shree Rejneesh, who believes that religious meditation is the answer to everything because the answers are within you, founded a center for religious meditation. This retreat in India is exceptionally popular with visitors of all nationalities and professions from all over the world. Today, there are about 600 different centers around the world.

• ***Maharishi Yogi***— Maharishi Majesh Yogi is an Indian monk who introduced to the world a very popular method of meditation known as transcendental meditation. His method is used by people who wish to reach an altered state of consciousness. His techniques include the art of breathing slowly, inhaling and exhaling, and using a mantra (which is the same word repeated over and over again) to help quieten the mind. This method is very popular among educators, especially doctoral students engaged in extensive research that calls for tremendous reading and recall.

SECTION 3
The Continuous Journey of Evolution and Kindness

1. Kindness and the Church of Scientology

With millions of followers throughout the world, The Church of Scientology is the church that stresses the ethics of goodness. Its doctrine is often considered more of a philosophy of life than a religion. Its teachings include religion, physics and science fiction. The founder, Ron Hubbard, author of *The Modern Science of Mental Health*, believed that unhappy events in our human lives can absorb our strength. But when we understand the roots of these unhappy events, the memory no longer controls us. In other words, we create our own reality and should, therefore, learn to cultivate kindness, love and compassion for one another and for ourselves for our own good mental health.

2. Kindness, Humility and the Philosophy of Cult Leaders

It has been said that most of today's religions were once-upon-a-time considered small cults. It is the practice of humility of the heart that made the difference. They adhered to the message of wisdom: "He that humbles himself shall be exalted."

The collective noun, "cult, is a term used for a group of people with similar beliefs. Cult is often associated with a guru.

Unfortunately, for the past few years, people have been very critical of cults because some gurus have let their egos take control instead of exercising humility, just as prophets before them have demonstrated. Jesus of Nazareth is the best example of kindness and humility. As the greatest teacher that ever lived, he has taught us by human examples to "follow him."

Many well meaning cult leaders have used their talents to abuse the spiritual profession. They have failed to catch the ego-thief or to conquer the ego. They failed to cultivate and live a life of humility from the heart.

Some gurus have been photographed or filmed enjoying lavish holiday vacations, driving fast and expensive automobiles and carelessly spending huge sums of money while preaching that their followers should live a simple life and give up their wealth. In our human life, when we achieve something, immediately pride, vanity and many other forces enter into our attitudes. We become overly excited and feel that the greatness comes from us, not knowing that our greatness is a direct line of creation from God through us to humanity. We "blow it" with the selfish ego.

Realizing that most of today's major religions were once small cults, we can imagine what would have happened if the leaders of our major religions had abused their leadership by becoming obsessed with self. While it is true that some fell by the wayside, we can meditate over the human experiences that caused them to fall and, like the weary traveler, ask for the spiritual message because God speaks to us through human experiences. The answer would probably be, "The experience is to teach you, my child. But you must be still and attentively listen to the inner voice with humility, kindness and understanding, in order to respond courageously to the experience with wisdom and knowledge." If we want to be kind and share our kindness with others and humanity, we have to cultivate a spirit of humility.

We learn from our great leaders who could have fallen by the wayside but did not because they were obsessed with the joy of following the God who created all things. These great leaders had found "the pearl of greatest price." They knew that fame and fortune would not bring eternal happiness. Only loving God and obeying His will can bring eternal joy that is everlasting.

When we really have something to offer and we want to offer it with a devoted quality, then humility automatically comes to the forefront. While we are achieving something, we have to constantly remember to be humble in order to be of greater service to mankind. In self-giving, we become truly happy.

The prophets have shown us that kindness makes us great, and when it is combined with the spirit of humility we become greater. God speaks to us through human experiences, commanding us to love one another and awakening us to transcendent wisdom and universal compassion.

3. Kindness is a Graceful Attitude of Serving Others

Caregiving experiences teach us that the purpose of our life is to give birth to the best attitude that is within us. Through gratitude journal writing, my husband and I learned this resurrection was our awakening.

We were awakened, through trials and tribulations of caregiver/patient relationships to realize that kindness is a graceful attitude to practice on a daily basis with everyone we encounter.

In cultivating the spirit of gracefulness, we must be careful about our choice of words when we extend help to others.

Caregiving experiences have taught me that we have to

be careful when we use the word "help." It would be better to use the word "service" instead, because when we serve someone, we have a feeling of humility. On the other hand, when we feel that we are helping someone, we oftentimes experience an attitude of pride, vanity and an ego that immediately surface. When we help someone, we feel that we have more capacity than someone else, and when we are being helped, we feel that we have less capacity. Implied by use of the word "help" there is a feeling of superiority or inferiority. But when we serve from the heart, there is no selfish pride because we do not feel superior. We feel that we are serving the Supreme in others. Fortunately, when we serve, we make the other person feel the presence of God within himself.

Caregiving experiences teach us that true service is always rendered with humility and kindness.

PART SIX
Kindness is the Cause of God in the World

It is only by the measure of thy humility that thou canst please God and save thyself, because it is certain that "God will save the humble of spirit."
— Fr. Cajetan Mary da Bergamo

Prelude

Finally and still athirst, the traveler asked, "Kind Master, how can the many religions teach me how to pray for a spirit of humility so that I can experience a life of inner peace while serving humanity with your spirit of kindness?"

And then the Master softly whispered, "My child, listen to dedicated lives of the prophets and the many faith founders, examine their spiritual attitudes of humility and kindness. They are there to teach you, my child, that kindness is the true religion."

Kindness is a Graceful Attitude of Humility

The great prophets and gurus who have exemplified dynamic leadership have shown us that if we wish to live in a world and work for a better world, our attitude should be one of dedicated service. We have been given a golden opportunity to serve others, and for this we should feel grateful to God.

When we feel that our ego is a thief inside us, denying us the opportunity to feel humble, we can chase it away through prayer and deep meditations just as, I am sure, our great prophets had to do. In the ego's purification and transformation is man's conscious evolution and true satisfaction.

We can conquer the ego and practice a graceful attitude of humility by using our imagination.

Suppose you are a great pianist and you are very proud of your artistic ability. Ask yourself whether you are the best pianist on earth. Your answer will be "no" because there are many who play the piano far better than you. No matter what we are proud of, we should ask ourselves whether there is anybody who is superior to us and our answer will always be "yes." We will find that there are many, many people whose skills are far better than ours in any aspect of life. Once we have awakened to this truth, how can we maintain our selfish pride?

Frankly, if we really want to rid ourselves of an inflated ego, vanity or pride, we can dive deep into the ocean of spiritual meditation. In so doing, we will be able to find our individual true selves and unlock our inherited divinity.

In our awakening to self-discovery, the ego cannot find a place to reside. When the spirit of peace, kindness, love, humility and joy come aboard, the egotistic feelings of vanity and pride will vanish. With this cleansing, we can enter into God's rest to love and to serve humanity as we, in meditation, embrace the following litany of humility.

A Litany of Humility to Cultivate the Spirit of Kindness

(Revised from *the Christian Action News*, "Spreading the word, Changing the World.")

Kind Master, in your lovingkindness, hear our prayer of humility that comes from the depths of our hearts...

From the desire of being praised, deliver us,
Kind Master.

From the desire of being honored, deliver us,
Kind Master

From the desire of being approved, deliver us,
Kind Master.

From the desire of being preferred, deliver us,
Kind Master.
From the desire of being esteemed, deliver us,
Kind Master.
From the desire of being loved, deliver us,
Kind Master.
From the desire of being extolled, deliver us,
Kind Master.
From the desire of being honored, deliver us,
Kind Master.

From the fear of being humiliated, deliver us,
Kind Master
From the fear of being suspected, deliver us,
Kind Master.
From the fear of being despised, deliver us,
Kind Master.
From the fear of being wronged, deliver us,
Kind Master.
From the fear of suffering rebukes, deliver us,
Kind Master.
From the fear of being ridiculed, deliver us,
Kind Master.
From the fear of being calumniated, deliver us,
Kind Master.
From the fear of being forgotten, deliver us,
Kind Master.

That others may be praised and I unnoticed, grant me
the grace, Kind Master.
That others may be chosen and I set aside, grant me
the grace, Kind Master.

That others may be preferred more than me, grant me
the grace, Kind Master.
That others may be lovedmore than I, grant me
the grace, Kind Master.
That others may be esteemed more than I, grant me
the grace, Kind Master.
That others may increase and I decrease, grant me
the grace, Kind Master.
That others become holier than I, as I become as holy
as I should, grant me the grace, Kind Master.

God Wants to be Kind Through Us

In summary, God wants to enter the world in us and through us; He wants to be *kind* through us. Kindness is the true religion. If we, as religious people, are not kind toward others, then they are tempted to be unkind like us. Then for them, there is no God because they do no see Him in us. The relation of their life to God is shattered by our behavior. Every unkind thing or action that we do to another person proves to him that there is no God. We all have the experience that the loss of a single soul can lead us to complete loneliness, disconnectedness, alienation, isolation, loss.

If we reject an individual or are unkind to him, we can make his world miserable and unhappy. As children of God, we have to be God's kindness so that others can recognize that kindness and love...lovingkindness...exist. And that despite everything, life is beautiful and good because God exists within us. It is through kindness that our life must become a "proof of God" for others. Man will reach God only through his brother. Love is kind.

Be kindly affectioned one to another with brotherly love.
— Romans 12:10.

The Spiritual Beauty of Kindness in Religions

National polls show that most people, especially family caregivers, believe in God and consider religion important in their lives. Spirituality, with its roots in kindness, is the fastest growing sector of the publishing industry, with millions of people buying books on the subject in search of healing techniques and inspiration.

But this rekindling of interest is not only a return to traditional religion. Over 32 million baby boomers, especially family caregivers, remain unaffiliated today, turning instead to Eastern practices, New Age philosophies, twelve Step programs, Greek mythology, Jungian psychology, shamanic practices, massage, yoga and a host of other traditions and practices. Many find spiritual fulfillment in music, poetry, literature, art, nature, intimate relationships and family caregiving. Many family caregivers find spiritual fulfillment in gratitude journal writing and poetry therapy.

Spirituality is now a major focus of the work of many psychologists. Although Freud believed that religion can be neurotic, and even those who are sympathetic to religion are reluctant to give it wholehearted approval, they confirm that religion does play some sort of role in one's mental health, but spirituality plays a major role. Carl Jung went so far as to say that spirituality was such an essential ingredient in psychological health that he could heal only those middle-age people who embraced a spiritual or religious perspective toward life.

The following are four basic ways to begin your spiritual journey into the world of kindness.

1. **Relaxation and Meditation.** On the segment of her daily talk show called "Remembering Your Spirit," Oprah Winfrey says that there is no greater source of strength and

power for her in life now than being quiet, meditating and recognizing what real power is.

2. **Prayer.** Prayer may indeed be the oldest spiritual practice and the most popular one in the world. Almost all world religions consider a form of it central to spiritual life. George Lucas, who plays on religious themes such as good and evil in his blockbuster Star Wars series, said that all religions are true. And that faith is a very important part of what allows us to remain stable and balanced. The emotional and mental release, along with a sense of connection to a transcendent dimension, goodness and universal compassion, may be at the heart of prayer's effectiveness.

3. **Spiritual Readings.** All of the world religions have writings which they consider sacred. Visit your library or local bookstore and browse around until you find something that speaks to you and is rich with suggestions. Football coach Mike Ditka says the Bible puts everything in perspective for him. For Mohammed Ali, the Qu'ran is the best "spiritual, building book." Bill Moyers text, *Healing and the Mind*, is a less traditional text that is used by talk show host Leeza Gibbons.

4. **Time in Nature.** We have all experienced powerful, spiritual moments when we have been confronted with earth's perfection and filled with awe. The author Henry David Thoreau tells us that nature was the temple of God and the perennial source of life for him when he fled civilization to live on Walden Pond. "The wind whips through the canyons of the American Southwest, and there is no one to hear it but us." Scientist Carl Sagan wrote as he spoke about his time-in-nature experience.

The Kindness Pledge

Family caregiving is a learning institution that teaches us the gift of kindness. It provides us with opportunities that show us how to be kinder to one another, even in difficult situations. When we pay greater attention to the things that we do and how we do them, we become more aware of even our most offhand daily actions. Through meditation and gratitude journal writing, we can find simple step-by-step and crucial spiritual directions on how to overcome the habitual unkindnesses that creep, undetected, into our caregiving behavior of even the more careful souls. It increases our insights into the wonders of the message that speaks so powerfully to us: "Love is patient, love is kind."

We, as family caregivers, can transform our world with kindness by devoting our lives to living the following pledge. This is a revised version of one given on a bookmark with research drawn from Lovasik's book, *The Hidden Power of Kindness: a practical handbook for souls who dare to transform the world, one deed at a time.* It is a pledge for family caregivers who want to make progress in the spiritual life that will enable them to live more fully with their loved ones and others, and more fruitfully in God's lovingkindness.

THE KINDNESS PLEDGE
FOR THE FAMILY CAREGIVER

As A Family Caregiver, I Resolve To:

(1) Speak kindly *of* my loved one and others.
(2) Think kindly *about* my loved one and others.
(3) Act kindly *toward* my loved one and others.
(4) Avoid speaking unkindly *of* my loved one or anyone.

(5) Avoid thinking unkindly *about* my loved one or anyone.
(6) Avoid acting unkindly *toward* my loved one or anyone.

Kindness is also known to be excellent holistic medicine because of its spiritual, mental and physical healing power. A Duke University study of 577 men and women hospitalized for physical illness showed that the more patients used positive religious coping strategies (seeking spiritual support from friends and religious leaders, performing deeds of kindness, having faith in God, meditating, praying) the lower the level of their depressive symptoms and the greater their quality of life.

Family caregiving experiences teach us that we can build a world of kindness. From the rain dances of Native Americans to the celebratory dances of Hasidic Jews, from the whirling dervishes of Islam to the meditating monks of Zen Buddhism, from the ecstatic worship service of charismatic churches to the solemn, silent meetings of the Quakers, spirituality takes on many kind expressions... because kindness is the true universal religion.

Epilogue

Feeling the gift of kindness within, the traveler entered her quiet space and lit a candle, quietly staring into its flame for an hour. Then slowly, she began to meditate on what her disabled brother had taught her about kindness through caregiving experiences.

Kindness within us, she learned, is a lighted candle of love.

Family caregiving experiences had taught her that when we have kind hearts, we have lighted candles that light our worlds where we meet God in our neighbor. Progress is in movement, and this movement comes when we feel the spirit of kindness within and use it to help transform the world, one kind deed at a time.

She learned that inasmuch as all of our world religions believe in the spirit of kindness, we must awaken to the awareness that it is spiritual to treat our neighbor kindly, whatever his faith, race, or nationality. As candlelights for the world, we should.

think with the spirit of kindness,
act with the spirit of kindness,
live with the spirit of kindness,
be the spirit of kindness.

And in the quietness of our souls, let us as a world, especially family caregivers, pray to our Eternal Father in harmony with our fellow travelers.

Heavenly Father,

As candlelights for the world of religions, we pray for those young souls, especially our young generation of tomorrow's leaders, who hear our sermons about kindness, who memorize our explanations of the meaning of life and do not feel our kindness nor our caring, concern or warmth. ...Kind Master, hear our prayer.

We pray for our nations that are fighting against one another rather than communicating peacefully in an effort to stop the unkindness and violence born of it against each other. ... Master of lovingkindness, hear our prayer

We pray for a new style of life, that we and all religious people throughout the world can be known by the kindness *and warmth of our caring and concern for one another. ...<u>Creator of all creation, in your lovingkindness, hear our prayer. Amen.</u>*

Spiritual Key # 4

Touching Lives, Lifting Spirits

"Inasmuch as anyone pushes you nearer to God, he or she is your friend."

FOREWORD
Candlelights and the Transformed Caregiver

I will give you a new heart and place a new spirit within you, taking from your bodies your stony hearts and giving you natural hearts.
Ezekiel 36: 26

Prelude

Searching for answers, a pilgrim stranger prayerfully asked, "Kind Master, I, too, am a family caregiver and You have said that my disabled brother is here to teach me kindness so that I can be a candlelight for the world. Today, how can I be awakened to this message in the midst of overwhelming responsibilities?"

The Kind Master replied, "My child, life speaks to you through your everyday experiences, enabling you to see that the past is history, the future is a mystery and today is a gift, that is why it is called the present. So light your candle and unwrap your present, and there you will find the spiritual message. But first you must be very quiet, meditate and listen attentively to your world."

1. The Message: Kindness is Spiritual/Caring

Family Caregiving, in my world, is a spiritual mission that enables us to find the Divine Life that lives within us and awakens us to the path of inner peace. When we share the caring, we find others who are kind and who can help us through stories that stir and nourish the soul. We also share messages that nourish the heart and body and inspirational meditations that help us to break through to the blessed, abundant life that the Creator has in store for us.

It is amazing to realize that when we reach out and perform

the extraordinary responsibilities of being a family caregiver with kindness, the Creator extends to us an extraordinary life of abundance to help us on the journey. Oftentimes we fail to see the hidden blessings, but when we exercise a spirit of patience, humility and gratitude, we encounter miracles that manifest His kindness and love.

Because we humans are interrelated, interconnected and interdependent, we need to be fully aware that our need for one another is a part of a Divine plan. When we isolate ourselves from others, we fail to see this spiritual blessing. We humans are a gift to one another, and as you and I experience life as family caregivers, we can readily see this truth in action.

Research tells us that, based on the amazing laws of cosmic mind power, man's thoughts become his abundance or his poverty. When we view our human experiences in the context of a loving plan, we can draw wisdom from them that can lead to the path of abundant life. On the other hand, when we isolate ourselves from the rest of humanity because of our selfishness, negative attitude or ingratitude, we deny ourselves the joy of loving, appreciating and respecting others and the joy of experiencing miracles.

The following section of this book relates to this fact of life. Family caregivers share a common bond regardless of the differences in their individual situations, and so the personal stories herein taken from my gratitude journals will provide a personal and heart-rending insight into family caregiving when we practice kindness, touch lives and lift spirits.

FOCUS ONE: AWAKENING

"God sends not ills when justly understood."

Through the eyes of God, my disabled husband saw a packed auditorium of eager listeners, but I, his heartbroken caregiver, saw only ten people surrounded by a huge pack of empty seats. Later, our gratitude journal writing revealed to us the entire experience and the spiritual awakening it provided.

It happened this way:

> Once upon a miracle, I was extended an invitation in November, 1998, to be a guest author at the Miami Book Fair International to read from my first book with my husband John entitled: *Mysterious Stranger Aboard: A Couple's Courageous 40-year Battle with Multiple Sclerosis*. The presentation would be part of the series, "Enhancing Our Lives: Exploring and highlighting the ties between mind, body and soul."
>
> My husband and I were overwhelmed with excitement for this invitation, which we considered a precious gift. At that time, I had no idea that ensuring experiences from this gift would pierce my heart. They would also teach me the wisdom of humility and gratitude yet again; show me that growth is painful and remind me that for every blessing there is a potential cross.
>
> John was even more excited than I because, according to the National MS Society, ours was the first book about multiple sclerosis written by patient and caregiver, and the book was being used by medical students at the Veterans Administration Hospital in

Miami in their MS research projects. In the book we had profiled the human experiences of our "triumphs over adversity, projecting our frustrations, depressions, exhaustion, anxiety, guilt, anger; our loss of privacy, future plans, economic security, health, family, friends and work."

He and I were delighted about my "fifteen minutes of fame," and I danced around his wheelchair doing the "Electric Slide," laughing into his laughter as we shared the good news. And then I wondered if there would be a crowd.

"John, sweetheart, I'm gonna ask God to help me pack that 500-seat Miami Dade Community College Auditorium with fans, just as He always helps me pack the 1,000-seat Joseph E. Caleb Auditorium and the 2,400-seat Dade County Auditorium with students who come to see our musical docudramas!"

John smiled and warned me to remain humble. Family caregiving is my passion, and I was quite exuberant about my invitation but I also listened to John. I tried to tone down the anxiety that was building.

Even so, I never expected the experience to be so painful. When I walked into the 500-seat auditorium and saw that only ten people had come to hear the reading, I inwardly shed silent tears.

A small voice inside my heart kept telling me to stop the silent crying because "the auditorium was filled to capacity." But the silent tears continued even as I listened attentively to the renowned Dr. Carlos Warter, a medical doctor and transpersonal psychotherapist who shared the platform with me. He talked dynamically about his books, The *Ebb and Flow of Living*; *Despertar; Soul Remembers*; and *Recovery of the Sacred*, a poignant and charming account of one man's journey along the road of self-discovery and fulfillment. Well now, those books sounded like the kind of wisdom that gratitude journal writing was offering John and me.

It seemed we shared a common bond of interest with Dr. Warter in touching lives and lifting spirits. When I made my presentation, he showed so much interest that I felt I was speaking to a packed audience. When he gave me his card and some literature about a project he was working on, I was shocked when I saw he was the co-author of a forthcoming book, *Chicken Soup for the Healing Soul.* The auditorium would have been packed had he used the bestselling "Chicken Soup for the Soul" title to promote his appearance. Everybody loves the *Chicken Soup for the Soul Series* because the books touch lives and lift spirits. I also realized that perhaps the auditorium would have been packed had I emphasized my seventh book, *Caring for the Caregiver*, because every caregiver wants to avoid caregiver-burnout. Of course the book also touches lives and lifts spirits.

But the thought of that empty auditorium agonized me for years. Nevertheless, amid the pain, I continued writing gratitude journals of family caregiving books.

And now, looking back on that experience, I can see it was preparing me for a time when our messages would pack rooms with people, I didn't realize this until years later, in late June, 2001, when I was in the midst of doing research on family caregiving for my twelfth book and looking for some *Chicken Soup for the Soul* books on the subject.

During that period, I was at the Veterans

Administration Medical Center nursing home reading to my husband *The Prayer of Jabez:*

And Jabez called on the God of Israel saying,
"Oh that You would bless me indeed, and enlarge
my territory, that Your hand would be with me,
and that you would keep me from evil,
that I may not cause pain!"
— 1 Chronicles 4:10 (NKJV).

"Chronicles 4:10?" I said, amazed. "John, sweetheart, your birthday is 4-10... April 10! And your name begins with 'J'. Jabez means pain; your MS is pain. It seems you and Jabez have lots of spiritual gifts in common. Jabez is a mysterious stranger that has come aboard. Folks say Jabez's prayer touches lives and lifts spirits, somewhat like the spiritual mission of your MS caregiving through gratitude journal writing has taught me!"

John chuckled and said, "Oh boy!" This simple response, I knew, was John's multipurpose response. Knowing that God answers the soul's attitude, he keeps his thoughts and words in a positive mode.

But, I was in for another mysterious surprise when I began reading interesting stories from *Chicken Soup for the Veteran's Soul.* In the first story, "Freedom Village," a Korean veteran gave flashbacks of his experiences during the Korean War. John had some of the same memories because he himself served in Korea at that time, and received an honorable discharge in 1953.

John enjoyed listening to these true stories published "to stir the pride and honor the courage of our veterans." They had touched his life and lifted his spirit so much that he said, "Family caregivers need chicken soup for their souls too, Alice." He suggested that I call the kind doctor from the Miami Book Fair International experience.

I gulped, then said sarcastically, "Frankly speaking, all I can remember is that frighteningly empty auditorium."

To this he quickly responded, "All you needed was the doctor who shared that podium with you. Alice." John implied that I should learn to be grateful and try to see God's creation in everything, in every aspect of my caregiving and his illness. He wanted me to always see that God has made all us humans to be interrelated, interconnected and interdependent. He knew our meeting was not coincidental, but a learning opportunity.

Adhering to my husband's metaphysical wisdom and author Bruce Wilkinson's faith-theory on *The Prayer of Jabez,* I rushed home, pulled Dr. Warter's brochures from the files and called the *Chicken Soup for the Soul* contact numbers. When I said that we need some "Chicken Soup for the Family Caregiver's Soul," I was told by a kind angel named "Valerie" to send her a proposal.

"What?" I shrieked, tears of joy clouding my eyes. "You mean to tell me authors Canfield and Hansen will consider publishing a book for the 54 million family caregivers out here who are crying for help? Wo-o-o-ow!" This was during the same week when a young Houston mother, who had been caregiving for her father with Alzheimer's disease, had drowned her five lovely children in the bathtub.

This shocking tragedy brought back my many memories of other tragic caregiving experiences. I saw the urgent need to submit a proposal for "Chicken Soup for the Family Caregiver's Soul" as an opportunity to enlarge our caregiving territory. "Oh that you would bless me indeed, and enlarge my territory." And, as a member of the National Family Caregivers Association, I would be honored to be considered as the book's co-author.

Days later, I received the application, quickly completed it and rushed it back.

Yes, with John's insight and encouragement, I now see thousands of packed "auditoriums of listeners" springing up from a seed that was planted November 17, 1998. The truth is, I do not have to be the main speaker because a collection of uplifting stories about the family caregiving experience will speak for itself to a world of suffering caregivers and their loved ones. With kindness, "God sends not ills when justly understood." He blessed John and me, indeed, and enlarged our territory.

I am grateful to *Chicken Soup for the Soul* Enterprises for its spirit of **kindness** and for *The Prayer of Jabez* and its illumination and inspiration. As a family caregiver, I especially appreciate a poem John and I had written for one of our musical docudramas projecting triumphs over adversity:

Let there be hope, rivers of hope where mortals will find love advening; Let there be hope, oceans of hope, where love will find its true meanings; Let there be hope, streams of great hope, where man's inhumanity to man can find its torture most demeaning!

2

Gratitude Journal Writing is Depression's Best Medicine.

Today, I carefully looked over the completed proposal for a book entitled *Chicken Soup for the Family Caregiver's Soul* which I mailed today to the publisher. Adhering to the application's guidelines, I included three (3) sample stories that I felt were representative of the proposed project, namely, stories from *Touching Lives, Lifting Spirits, Caring for the Caregiver* and *Mysterious Stranger Aboard.* Strangely enough and without giving it a second thought at the time, I quickly excerpted an edited copy of Chapter One from the manuscript, "Caring for the Caregiver," as though some higher force was controlling my thoughts and actions.

What actually amazed me is that the opening story fit perfectly with the proposal project. I was dumbfounded.

When I was writing this story in my gratitude journal in 1997, I was depressed and was writing through the pain of what had actually happened, reliving every minute of it. When I finished the entire book, I actually felt spiritually healed because the writing was spiritual psychotherapy.

A study conducted by Dr. David Antonuccio, a psychologist at the Reno, Nevada, Veteran's Administration Medical Center, found that psychotherapy works as well as or better than medication to treat depression.

For my husband and me, gratitude journal writing is an excellent form of psychotherapy. It includes cognitive therapy, which changes the way family caregivers and their care recipients think about events in their lives; and interpersonal therapy, which changes how family caregivers and their care recipients interact with others.

The following is a chapter I included in the proposal:

CARING FOR THE CAREGIVER

By Alice W. Johnson

"Depressed, Nurse Pinkney pulled the trigger and ...Bang! Bang! Bang! The blood of her disabled, wheelchair-bound husband with multiple sclerosis, and the blood of her two beautiful kids splattered all over the kitchen, Alice!" my husband's 58-year-old mother had tearfully said to me that early-spring morning of 1973. "And, Alice, those sweet little innocent kids were only 3 and 5," she added sadly, "and 'er husband was my precious little John's age."

I was weeping also, shaking my head and staring into Cincinnati, Ohio, blue skies, bepuzzled. I did not know at that time that, according to research, family caregivers experience depression more than the rest of the population, and that I would be a victim of this same kind of experience if I did not seek help.

Earlier, we both had been compassionately talking about John, my 41-year-old scholarly husband and her only son, who was just diagnosed with multiple sclerosis (sometimes called MS) a week earlier. We were discussing how the MS symptoms first appeared in 1952 while he was stationed in Korea, and we were wondering why didn't the army medical professionals recognize his on-and-off stumbling and falling.

As I now sit writing in my gratitude journal, a therapeutic activity suggested by talk show hostess Oprah Winfrey as a "self-help" focus, how painfully I recall my disabled husband's mother (whom I called Mom) telling me about the frightening Nurse Pinkney story as we worked in the flower garden planting tulips. She was shaking with sobs and I had moved to embrace her.

Mom was a head nurse at Drake Memorial Hospital in Cincinnati. Through stifling tears, she told me of her twenty-eight-year-old, beautiful, blonde co-worker, Nurse Pinkney, who had killed her entire family—her husband and two children—the previous day out of caregiver's frustrations and depressions. Because she knew that the universe speaks to us through human experiences, Mom prayerfully begged me to see the spiritual message of that tragedy and to get spiritual help for John and me as quickly as possible.

"Remember, Alice, attitude is everything," she warned. "So try to always keep a spiritual attitude because everything is in God and God is in everything."

"Wow!" I said with awe. "Frankly, Mom, I don't understand your motherly wisdom so I'll leave that alone. Besides, John and I are both very religious!" Mom quickly responded, " But so were the Pinkneys, Alice."

I had gulped, then said with humility and compassion, "Well, Mom, because you whispered a mother's prayer, I'm sure we'll keep in mind your fervent request."

She clutched both my shoulders and her watery eyes stared piercingly into mine, "Please take care of each other. I love both of you very much."

Nine months later, on March 8, 1974, Mom died unexpectedly in a diabetic coma. For a time we wept unceasingly, feeling that the stress of John's illness and the fear that I would suffer caregiver-burnout and harm him had contributed to her early demise. We wept even harder, remembering all that she had taught us about being spiritually strong so that we could triumph over adversity and make our lives productive.

Seven months following her death, on December 18, 1974, John and I moved to the beautiful, "magic city" of Miami, Florida to begin a new chapter in our turbulent life with MS. We purchased a lovely home in the suburbs. I retired from my teaching position and became a full-time family caregiver for him.

Although we were warmly received into Miami's society, I felt disconnected and isolated because the stress of caregiving was mounting along with John's debilitating illness; and we were too ashamed to share our thoughts and feelings. We thought about Mom's prayer and her fear that we might be driven to emulate Nurse Pinkney's episode. Then immediately, we both sought help. It was our analyst, Dr. Jack W. Kensinger, along with our family physician, Dr. John T. McAdory, and the memory of the Pinkney family tragedy that saved us from the disasters of caregiver and patient-burnout.

Adhering to our doctors' professional counseling, we took charge of our lives. Because we were former school teachers with a passion for sharing knowledge, we founded Mal-Jonal Productions, Inc., a non-profit organization, and began writing and producing musical docudramas for children, emphasizing multicultural education and literacy. The docudramas portrayed positive role models who had triumphed over adversity. Writing was excellent therapy for the two of us; so we went on a writing spree.

Flashing back into the chain of events, I now

guessed that no one had actually told Nurse Pinkney that family caregiving is a spiritual mission in which most of us caregivers strive for faithfulness, sanity and inner peace rather than sainthood. This message was a spiritual blessing my husband and I fully discovered through deep meditations and counseling, and after writing about our thoughts, feelings and emotions in our daily gratitude journals. Undoubtedly, it was the spiritual message John's mother had reference to regarding the Pinkneys' incident. "Trust life and it will teach you."

In our first self-styled journal, *Mysterious Stranger Aboard* (MS Aboard) which was published in 1996, we projected our 40-year battle with MS, our frustrations, depressions, exhaustion, anxiety, guilt, anger; and our loss of privacy, future plans, economic security, health, family, friends, and work. The book showcases the suffering we endured with the crippling disease that saps motor skills made worse by the aftermath of Miami's 1992 Hurricane Andrew that blew John into the Veterans Administration Medical Center nursing home and blew me deeper into his MS world, to awaken the spirit of kindness and the inherited divinity within both of us.

Frustrations mounted, John's deteriorating illness mounted, and our gratitude journal writing and understanding mounted, sending us to higher levels of spiritual growth. By gratitude journal writing through the pain, and being joyfully engaged in creating and producing cultural activities to help heal humanity, we were gradually awakened to the world of love, kindness and compassion. Through caregiving experiences, we were awakened to the wisdom that all creation is holy, even the suffering, sickness, pain and death that we all experience here on planet earth.

We accept good things from God; and should we not accept evil? — Job 2:10b

We thought about the Pinkneys' experiences, and we thought about our own as caregiver and patient. We realized that even my husband's multiple sclerosis was holy and is here to teach us humans through caregiving examples that kindness is the truest religion. "Kindness stops the torrent of angry passion, takes the sting from failure and kindles courageous ambition."

Because the Pinkneys' tragedy has shown us by extension the importance of caring for the caregiver with love, kindness and compassion, John and I have made "Caring for the Family Caregiver" our spiritual ministry. In memory of the Pinkneys, all of our creative writings are geared to spread the news to others that caregiving is a spiritual mission that enables us to help cultivate the spirit of love, kindness and compassion for all humanity. When we view all life's experiences in the context of a loving plan, this understanding constitutes the greatest source of spiritual strength imaginable.

And now, I am sitting here tearfully meditating, still amazed at how mysteriously and quickly I included the above chapter in the proposal. Somehow, I feel very strongly that the spirit of Mom, along with those of Mr. Pinkney and his two children, had chosen it for me.

3

Those who bring the spirit of love and compassion to the lives of others cannot keep it from themselves.

Today, I visited my husband at the VA Hospital Medical Center. Still somewhat mesmerized by the thought of loving spirits mysteriously pulling that particular chapter on family caregiving from the hundreds of chapters we have written on the subject, I told him about the strange feeling.

He smiled and agreed that my intuition could be correct.

Then, in his stammering speech he tried to tell me that the mystery was a direct line of creation from God through me to the book proposal committee because I have a passion for caring for the caregivers and their loved ones.

I said the experience proved there was another mysterious stranger aboard on our lives' journey.

Frankly, I am beginning to believe that the spirit of caregiving itself is a "mysterious stranger aboard" as well, because it teaches us that when we bring blessings into the lives of other people, we cannot keep them from ourselves. I still feel exceptionally good about the possibility of us family givers generating some "chicken soup" for each other's souls. When my husband slowly asked me what other sample story did I send, I told him *Mysterious Stranger Aboard.*

When he asked me what chapter, I told him an edited version of Chapter One. I suppose he thought I had submitted the chapter he had written about his experience in the Korean War.

Perhaps I could have sent that chapter, but the other was more representative of the proposed project because it dealt with family caregiving and care receiving. This, too, was a mystery because I had mysteriously pulled the chapter and had hurriedly shortened it.

Why was I rushing? Because when the application arrived, my intuition told me to quickly complete it and rush it back because electrical thunderstorms and flooding were predicted for our area. Florida's lightning oftentimes strikes and kills. Perhaps I was paranoid about the windstorm, so I included a chapter about Hurricane Andrew that had to do with the tedious responsibilities of caregiving for a loved one during crisis situations. I had to shut down my computer before the lightning shut it down for me.

The following is the shortened chapter I hurriedly included. As I was retyping and shortening it, I felt that I was reliving the terrifying experience it describes while the spirit of my now-deceased sister and mentor, Jessye, who played a major role in this event when she was alive, guided my fingers across the keys. It was she who had begged me to evacuate because of the hurricane, and I had waited too late.

MYSTERIOUS STRANGER ABOARD
by Alice and John Johnson

Then the Lord answered Job out of the whirlwind:
"Have the gates of death been opened unto thee?
Or has thou seen the doors of the shadow of
death?" (Job 38:1,17)

God is life; to love other people is to see His face. Prior to this perception, my husband and I were sinking in our doubts about accepting this truth, and it took a mysterious stranger, multiple sclerosis to come aboard and throw us a lifeline that being our brother's keeper humanizes us all, and gives us the "high" we all seek.

I was considering this insight, lost in silent thought, when the telephone's apologetic jingle startled me.

My husband John, a 40-year victim of a chronic disease that robs motor skills, laid his editing pencil on the desk and with his paralyzed left hand, lifted the receiver to his ear and spoke softly, then listened intently. Had I known this would be the last accurate conversation he would have, I would have been far more serious about evacuating for the hurricane. And I might also have missed the tremendous lesson that ultimately awakened me to John's oft-repeated wisdom that "God is life."

My husband continued talking into the phone, now shaking his head and laughing heartily. "OH, No-o-o-o! We don't think our Hurricane Andrew will be as disastrous as your Hurricane Hugo was! No way! But the Miami Herald reports that it might be "THE BIG ONE!"

Following a period of listening, he continued. "Yes, we've been told that Hurricane Andrew's scheduled to be here tomorrow night; but shucks...here in Miami, we've been threatened with hurricanes before." His voice was gentle, his slurring speech pronounced. "So, my Alice and I will pray, as usual, and follow the media's advice. She's a good caregiver. But, oh boy! this morning the media reported that tropical storm Andrew is now a hurricane headed directly at South Florida, about 800 miles east of Miami with winds a little over 75 mph. That guy's a son-of-a-gun!"

It was August 22, 1992, and the two o'clock sun made quirky leaf patterns against white sheer curtains in the office of our South Dade suburban home. News reports of Hurricane Andrew flowed from the radio-intercom. Although terrified, I was determined to hide my fears from John to control the stress he might encounter and which could be detrimental to his remaining health.

"Turn the sound down, Alice" he said, his hand covering the receiver. His neatly trimmed salt and pepper hair made him look distinguished, as usual.

I lowered the sound and continued editing our life story on the Macintosh LCII. It would be the first life story written by caregiver and patient. Listening to his telephone responses, I knew it was my older sister, Jessye, from Sumter, South Carolina, on the line. She had been a victim of Hurricane Hugo and was anxious to help us survive Andrew and its aftermath, just as she survived Hugo.

Yesterday, Jessye and my oldest sister, Georgia, had called and said that Hugo started out as a tropical depression in the South Atlantic. Hugo hit the southeast coast of the United States at Charleston, South Carolina, on September 21, 1989. It killed several people and cost seven billion dollars in damage. And now my sisters wanted us to evacuate because Hurricane Andrew could be another Hurricane Hugo. Feeling a strong sense of security at that time, I told them the news media said that those of us living west of US-1 did not have to evacuate.

Jessye was hysterical. "Listen, Alice," she had said, "if YOU feel secure enough not to evacuate, then, as your husband's caregiver, GET JOHN TO A SHELTER, PLEASE! Call the Veterans Administration Center NOW and get John out of that house BEFORE IT'S TOO LATE! God has entrusted you with John's care!"

Well, now it was too late because VA had

repeatedly announced that it would be picking up veterans until Saturday noon. Already it was past 2 P.M. I listened as John continued talking into the phone.

"Well, Jessye," he said, cheerfully, "I used to wonder what's the meaning of life that the inevitability of death doesn't destroy? My experiences of being in the Korean War and my experiences with this disease have revealed the answer. LOVE. Love is the purpose of life; God is life. All creation is holy, even Hurricane Andrew." He smiled, said his "thanks for calling us," then handed the phone to me.

I stared at him wide-eyed, nodding my head because I, too, wanted to *feel* that God is life. "John, aren't you gonna finish editing our life story?" I asked, my right hand covering the receiver.

"No, Alice, I'm going to the family room and watch the news reports on the big screen. Just as your sister warned, according to news reports this hurricane's gonna be monstrous!"

"But, John, our editor is waiting for *Mysterious Stranger Aboard.* We're already behind schedule," I said, knowing that writing always keeps us calm and peaceful.

"Alice, with Hurricane Andrew threatening, we can expect another mysterious stranger aboard!" he said seriously, steering his wheelchair toward the family room.

Jessye and I talked for a split second, long enough to put the scare in me as an unthinking, confused caregiver at such a crucial time as this.

Now terribly frightened, I tried to call VA but could not get through. "Dear God, please help me!" I prayed silently. "Please forgive me for being a lousy caregiver. I should have taken my husband to a shelter." I felt frustrated, confused, depressed. "I need help!"

Undoubtedly, the Creator heard my fervent prayer because immediately two of our kind male neighbors came over and offered to help prepare our house for the hurricane. They pulled our hurricane shutters over the windows and doors, secured the pool patio and back porch furniture. John and I were very grateful. He and I had already stocked our kitchen pantry with emergency goods and had taken care of other necessities, even though we're often threatened with hurricanes that do not come.

The media kept announcing that those of us who lived on the west side of US-1 did not have to evacuate. We were innocently trusting the media, just as we Miamians have always trusted the wisdom of our meteorologists.

On Sunday morning, Andrew was strengthening and heading for South Florida. When we heard "Category 4," we knew it was very bad news. At 8 p.m., the National Hurricane Center announced that the storm was 185 miles east of Miami and described it as "extremely dangerous." I prepared John for bed, tucked him in, then hurried back to the computer. At 12:13 a.m. Monday, meteorologist Bob Sheets' voice bounced from the TV, "It looks more like it's coming right across South Dade! The storm is staying on course, moving like a locomotive on steel tracks headed directly for South Dade!"...the part of the county in which we lived.

"Good Heavens!" I shrieked, jerking the disc from the computer. Quickly, I grabbed the edited manuscript from John's desk, and snatched the Holy Bible from the library shelf. With the Bible and fifteen years of tedious research pressed to my heart, I hurried to the bedroom where I found John fast asleep.

Staring nervously at the bedroom TV screen and listening to gushing winds sounding like a freight train plowing into our house, I chanted John's mantra, "God is Life," but could not cease trembling. I listened as TV meteorologist Bryan Norcross told us listeners what to do and what not to do.

According to the 3 a.m. news report, 140-mph winds were now 40 miles east of Miami. Suddenly the lights went out and I hurriedly found Norcross' voice on the radio, snatched the flashlight from the nightstand and fell to my knees saying "God is life. God is life. Please forgive me for not taking my husband to a shelter!" even amid the roaring thunder and flashing lightning; even as the terrified voice on the radio thundered, "Hurricane Andrew's eye-wall has roared ashore in South Dade!" Yes, the gates of death had opened unto us and we saw the doors of the shadow of death.

Insulation from the ceiling blew into my face. I jumped up from the floor, awakened John, helped him in the wheelchair and whisked him to the walk-in clothes closet. A split-second later the ceiling collapsed on the bed. I was panic-stricken, but a voice inside me kept saying "God is life and life is God. His life is in you."

"Why aren't you afraid, John?" I screamed above the roaring sounds of Andrew, hurriedly tucking him inside the closet and fearing that we both were going to die.

He squeezed my trembling hand and said above the sound of gushing winds, "Alice, I'm accustomed to foxholes. The army taught us that God is everywhere, in everything and everything is in Him. Try to feel His life within you."

It was then that I realized that John *felt* deep within what he was saying, and there is a difference between knowing and *feeling*. I wanted so badly to feel the love but I was frightened beyond words. The only feeling I was feeling was fear. If God sounded anything like His angry thunder and lightning, I felt totally helpless.

Suddenly flashes of lightning streaked, followed immediately by a long, boisterous roar of thunder. Others followed within seconds and John suggested that I keep asking for inner peace. I did, even as I heard the roof being blown off the house and angry winds breaking glass and tossing furniture everywhere. I wondered how did our trusted meteorologists misguide those of us who lived on the west side of US-1. John sensed my fears and said above the sound of howling winds, "Alice, try to *feel* love in your body, mind, heart and soul; and be convinced of eternal life! Just as light is the opposite of darkness, love is the opposite of fear!"

Mysteriously, while adhering to my husband's wisdom, it seemed a light abruptly turned on inside me and I began to feel the joy of love and peace within. My fears subsided and I fell asleep not knowing that this was the last accurate and articulate conversation he would have.

Four hours later, we awakened into the silver-gray morning of August 24, 1992, to discover that

Hurricane Andrew had totally destroyed South Dade, including our home. Staring into the piles of debris, we found it difficult to believe that we were alive.

Miraculously, only 38 deaths directly related to the hurricane were reported in South Florida, where over 45 million people reside. However, Hurricane Andrew was the worst disaster ever to befall the United States. Its grim toll totaled $20 billion in damages.

As a result, a tremendous outpouring of love and service came from all over the world! In the midst of all this love, kindness and compassion for one another, we saw the face of God. It was the most beautiful *feeling of unconditional love* one could ever experience. It was the kind of spiritual feeling that experiences of family caregiving offer us as a divine gift.

In more human terms, over 63,000 homes were destroyed (most of them in South Dade, especially west of US-1), and over 100,000 were damaged. Over 250,000 people were left homeless; John and I were among them. The Veterans Administration Medical Center moved quickly to place him in the nursing home. He was a medical victim of Andrew's aftermath due to a series of flare-ups that increased the severity of his disability.

The murderous windstorms of Hurricane Andrew blew us into the beautiful world of gratitude journal writing, awakening us to transcendent wisdom, universal compassion and inner peace. On the journey, our human experiences taught us by example that God is life; and to love one another is to see His face.

This unforgettable experience happened almost nine years

ago. And now it is again August, and the weather outside is very stormy.

Over the years, gratitude journal writing has given us the key to life and inner peace. It has taught us to be thankful, to be fully aware and observant of the many, many people who are forever touching our lives and lifting our spirits. Hurricane Andrew taught us by example the wisdom of the old-age adage: "It's an ill wind that blows no good."

Yes, Andrew, though destructive, blew lots of good to many of us South Floridians.

Prior to Hurricane Andrew, many of our beautiful houses were badly in need of major repairs that would cost us fortunes, but the home insurance companies had smart executives who knew how to quickly find legitimate reasons to evade the issues. Even our membership in the Home Owners Association could not make them bulge. So, our home insurance companies paid nothing.

Our house needed a new roof, and when our home insurance company denied our claim, we had to pull thousands of dollars out of our puny savings to replace the roof. Then Andrew came two months later and blew the darn thing off along with 63,000 other home roofs. We wanted to sue Mother Nature for child abuse, but we were too blessed to be stressed. In all seriousness, we were blessed to be alive!

Although unknown to John, he and I were on the verge of going bankrupt. Yes, John and I were encountering financial woes because of the high medical expenses that stemmed from his disability. The Veteran's Administration was doing hardly anything to help us, and it kept denying him compensation for his service-connected disability, knowing that his MS symptoms flared up when he was in the Korean War. The Internal Revenue showed no mercy that John could no longer cut the huge lawn or assist with property upkeep, and that we had to pay heavily for assistance, minor home repairs, and all the many expenses that can create caregiver-burnout. For this reason, we were fighting very hard to stay afloat physically, spiritually, financially, and productively.

Yes, our beautiful house was totaled, but we received full coverage that saved us from the prison of bankruptcy. My analyst told me to use John's economic wisdom in managing wisely the monies we received from our home insurance company.

Following the analyst's counseling, I did what John would have done. With continuous prayer, gratitude and humility, I paid off the home mortgage after rebuilding our home, paid off all debts and put the balance of the money in savings.

With VA caring for John, we were able to continue writing and producing musical docudramas emphasizing multicultural education and literacy, in our endeavor to be productive. The Cultural Affairs Council and the Board of County Commissioners awarded us many grants to continue bringing our cultural talents to the Miami community. In spite of the monstrous Hurricane Andrew, we South Miamians survived with the help of the Creator and rebuilt South Dade, making the entire district attractive and scenic, especially our spiritual lives.

John, in spite of his inability to speak clearly and in complete sentences, has often joked that "Maybe we should have sued Mother Nature for child abuse" when we think about this chapter in our lives. Caregiving has taught us that good humor makes all things bearable.

"Knowing our surviving that hurricane was absolutely a miracle from the Creator, we are grateful to be alive and for the beautiful, spiritual world we have discovered through gratitude journal writing.

4

Wisdom from Hurricane Andrew

"It's an ill wind that blows no good."

John and I wrote a poem of gratitude immediately following Hurricane Andrew's onslaught, projecting how it touched lives and lifted spirits. Surprisingly, the poem was broadcast on national TV as the media showed scenes of Andrew's destruction one year later. Friends were calling us from all over the country, telling us that they saw my picture on national TV as I dramatically read a poem while terrifying scenes from Hurricane Andrew's murderous windstorm ran in the background.

In our gratitude journal writing about the hurricane, we found the hidden power of kindness and compassion as people from all over the world reached out to help touch lives and lift spirits.

ABOUT HURRICANE ANDREW
(August 24, 1993)

Once upon a hurricane, 'twas just one year ago,
Mid-summer, nineteen hundred ninety-two,
Saint Andrew blew away our world that August twenty-four
Exposing all our cobwebs and mildew.

We wept but for a moment, then we started to rebuild
Though frustrations mounted everywhere;
We wrestled with anxieties of contracts unfulfilled
As love and wisdom filled the atmosphere.

The doors of our spirits were awakened to this call
And love's bright light of wisdom came aboard;

We pushed aside our egos and our selfish iron-walls
Then saw within ourselves love's great award.

The wisdom of compassion, love and sharing filled our hearts
As we embraced each victim of the storm;
The flow of love that came from us was nature's work of art
We never dreamed that love could be so strong.

Love always finds expression through its kindness and concern
And Andrew gave us opportunities
To love and help each other; Andrew's lesson we had learned
As we embraced our multi-culturalness.

We learned the art of loving, patience, kindness, gratitude
As we embraced them with humility;
We learned the joy of loving with a caring attitude
That gives us all respect and dignity.

We've learned that our Creator is indeed both cause/effect
And love's the greatest creation of life;
Andrew taught us love's wisdom; an award we all respect,
A blessing from St. Andrew's calm and strife.

Wisdom has taught us that we are created with love's gift
But our egos were smothering this view
And our Creator, caring, saw us selfishly adrift
Then spoke to us through Hurricane Andrew.

An attitude of gratitude has led us to the light
That helping one another is what counts
And saying "thank you" to our helpers is a satellite
That brings us happiness in huge amounts.

From all around the world the blessings came, to our surprise,
In kind symbols of love from everywhere;
We learned that our Andrew was a blessing in disguise,
And that his message was a godsent prayer.

We are interconnected with each other on this plane;
To spread love is our purpose, we have learned;
We are interdependent and it took a hurricane
To teach us love with kindness and concern.

We're grateful to Saint Andrew for the message that he brought
And grateful for abundant blessings, too;
We thank the world of people and the lessons that it taught
That we are vessels; and we thank Andrew.

An Addendum:

So-o-o-o-o...
By touching lives and lifting spirits we answer the call
To be vessels of love to one another;
God speaks to us through our experiences as He tells us all
To touch lives and lift spirits of each other.

Yes, Hurricane Andrew has taught us that kindness is the true religion because when we are kind, we touch lives and lift spirits. Writing in my self-created style of gratitude journaling, I am able to reflect on hundreds of magnificent miracles in which I have seen the spirit of kindness exemplified. Writing a proposal for a "Chicken Soup for the Soul" book, after reading several of the books in the series, has shown me that kindness is indeed one of God's greatest gifts to the world. With this inspiration, I feel a passion for now completing a manuscript I have been anxiously writing entitled *Kindness is the True Religion.*

Unfortunately, I cannot work on the book today because I

have to attend the funeral of one of my loving sorority sisters who died suddenly and unexpectedly on the same day I was executing my proposal. She would have been so delighted that I was asked to submit a proposal for a "Chicken Soup for the Soul" book on family caregiving. Ironically, I had looked forward to sharing the good news with her later on the same day she died. She had a passion for books and was a board member of Miami Book Fair International. She also was the vice-president of our Miami Alumnae Chapter of Delta Sigma Theta Sorority, Inc., and an excellent board advisor for the sorority committee which I chaired—Arts and Letters.

Her personality was the perfect example of human kindness, love and compassion. Although I am badly shaken by her sudden death, my intuition tells me to finish the manuscript on" "kindness" to be shared with other family caregivers before another monstrous hurricane like Andrew blows into Miami. Perhaps it is her spirit speaking into my sadness. If so, I have grown accustomed to the experience of spirits of love directing my fingers, as most writers can attest.

5

Our true blessings oftentimes appear to us in the shape of disappointment and pain.

Today, we are experiencing lots of rain, and Tropical Storm Barry has intensified to near-hurricane strength and is threatening Miami. And because we see no lightning just now, I can let my fingers dance across computer keys in our home office and write through feelings of disappointment and pain that are attempting to surface because of the sudden death of my girlfriend's husband. She, too, was a family caregiver for her disabled husband who served in the Korean War.

Today, through gratitude journal writing, I feel the need

to bring into focus all the many people and their programs that are touching lives and lifting spirits because they know that we are here on earth to serve God and to fulfill Him. What a joyful mission for the soul; it enhances happiness and inner peace.

The *Chicken Soup for the Soul* series is sharing its wisdom with John and me in so many areas of personal growth and interest. For this we are truly grateful. There is nothing more entertaining than pensively listening to experiences that project the miracle of human kindness.

Yesterday, John had asked what was the third sample story I had sent with the proposal. I told him that it was not about his experience in Korea. Rather, it was about his seeing a full auditorium through the eyes of God when he learned that a co-author of a proposed "Chicken Soup for the Soul" book was sharing the stage with me, and my seeing an empty auditorium through my human eyes.

He had laughed, then implied that Mysterious Stranger's (his MS) wisdom had seen the packed auditorium with an agenda to reach out and help millions of others. I told him that illnesses like MS always come with wisdom...because wisdom is born in suffering; and caregiving experiences have shown us that suffering is a gift.

Oops! It's lightning, so I must quit here and continue later. Miami's lightning is known to strike people and their computers. Fortunately, I have learned the joy of meditating in my quiet space while Miami's boisterous thunderstorms are raging. It is an excellent time to reflect on one's thoughts and feelings to promote spiritual growth.

6

It's almost midnight and Tropical Storm Barry has flirted

with us as most of his relatives have done in the past. My intuition tells me to resume writing my thoughts and feelings, and I will get clarification about this emotional unrest.

This morning, when I visited my husband at the VA Medical Center Nursing Home to take him to Mass, I was shocked to be told that he has pneumonia. He had just recovered from the same illness a month ago. I noticed that when I returned home this evening, I went directly to the computer in an attempt to write through the pain, as usual. Now that I have meditated with my higher self, and Tropical Storm Barry has jilted us, I can talk bravely about today's experiences.

This morning, I attended the 8 A.M. mass at Christ the King Catholic Church as usual, sang in the choir, then drove the twenty-five miles to VA to join John at their 10:45 A.M. mass service.

" Mrs. Johnson, we did not get your husband out of bed this morning because he has pneumonia," the nurse kindly said when I entered the nursing home unit.

"What?" I asked, anxious to rush to his bedroom with my briefcase filled with **Chicken Soup for the Soul** books to later read to him more good stories that touch lives and lift spirits. "How could he get pneumonia overnight?"

"Last night he was wheezing and had a difficult time breathing," the nurse replied, "so we had the doctor check him. When the test results came back, they showed pneumonia."

"What?" I again asked, dumbfounded. And now this family caregiver needed some chicken soup for *her* soul. Even though I was no stranger to this kind of experience as a family caregiver, and that my response is what we caregivers call anticipatory grief, I still needed some chicken soup for my soul. It would give me more spiritual and moral support at a time like this. Reading about the human experiences of other family caregivers would have made me feel more interconnected, interdependent and interrelated, just as John felt about the veterans' stories.

Touching lives and lifting spirits is what *Chicken Soup for the Soul* does at a time like this. So, I had my husband's holistic medicine packed in my briefcase ready to administer it to him. Luckily, he always enjoys hearing the stories from *Chicken Soup for the Veteran's Soul* because veterans, like family caregivers, share a common bond regardless of the differences in their individual situations.

"Hi, sweet baby!" I whispered after entering his room, standing by his bedside and kissing him on the forehead.

"Hi!" he responded, the IV apparatus making its tick-tick sound as he was being given antibiotics intravenously.

"How do you feel, sweetheart?" I smiled, staring at the huge green oxygen tank with its long, thin tube extended around my husband's ears and slowly feeding oxygen into his nostrils.

"Fine," he said, unsmiling.

Then pulling a book from the briefcase, I said gleefully. "Look, John, sweetheart, I brought you some delicious '"chicken soup" for your "veteran's soul!"

His eyes lit up and he chuckled. "Oh boy, *Chicken Soup for the Veteran's Soul.*"

"Good chicken soup, John!" I said with enthusiasm. "Chicken soup to stir the pride and honor the courage of you wonderful veterans!"

"Wow!" he said, his eyes aglow. "Read about Korea?"

"There's one in here called "Christmas in Korea" by Larry Ebsch. He talks about how he and his buddies jumped in their ambulance and visited the kids at the orphanage; taking them Spam, crackers, cookies, candy, gum and all kinds of wrapped

Christmas presents. He tells how happy the kids and the nuns were!"

"Wow!" my husband said with stretched, smiling eyes.

Just as I was about to comfortably sit down and begin reading the story to John, the x-ray technician entered with his huge machine. And behind him was a cute little "Nurse Dracula" who came to draw John's blood.

My intuition told me to leave the room and attend the VA Mass in the chapel while the medical staff performed their responsibilities.

Quickly, I kissed John's forehead, told him I was going to mass and would return later, then made an exit.

Accepting the unexpected

As I was leaving the room enroute to mass my good friend, Cammie, met me in the hallway, clutched both my shoulders and said softly, "Alice, my husband has gone back to God. He died peacefully early this morning."

"What?" I exclaimed, staring sadly into watery-smiling eyes. The four of us...Cammie and husband, John and me... were always together enjoying the company of each other. Both men are war veterans, Catholics, former school teachers with doctorate degree in education and creative writers. Cammie and I are both very active Catholics and family caregivers who are supportive of our husbands. We caregiving wives have an unusual bond. We live with anticipatory grief that has made us spiritually strong. We feel this is a part of the Master's loving plan that promotes spiritual growth.

"Yes, he died softly," Cammie said. " On yesterday, he appeared so peaceful and happy. Smiling at everyone. And now he has slipped away to return to God. Come inside the room and see him."

Compassionately, I entered the room and stood by the

bed where her husband laid as though he were peacefully sleeping, as usual. I made the sign of the cross and touched his cold hands as I whispered a prayer, thanking him for making his life a blessing to others by spreading love and kindness to help heal the world. Then, with my forefinger, I made a cross on his forehead, thanking the Creator for His gift of love...Cammie's wonderful husband. Other family members were present.

Cammie had a healthy attitude about death; an attitude she had learned from the experiences of being a family caregiver.

Just last Sunday I had given Cammie a copy of the magazine entitled: *Pope John Paul II Life: A Tribute* by Robert Sullivan and the editors of *Life*. She spoke of how much her husband loved the interesting photographs and the story.

And now I must give Cammie's grieving family members a copy of *Chicken Soup for the Christian Family Soul* because its stories open the heart and rekindle the spirit at a time like this.

After giving Cammie and her family bear hugs, I told Cammie that I was en route to the chapel and would see her when I return. She told me that she was going to mass also, as soon as Father Damian arrived to give her husband his last rites.

En route to the VA chapel, I met Father Damian rushing to Cammie's husband's room. He suggested that I, as a lecturer for the mass, continue to the chapel and help get the necessities set up for him so that we could proceed on schedule.

Amazingly, everything at the mass service worked out beautifully, peacefully, perfectly and on schedule and I knew that God, as usual, was in total control. As a reader for the mass, I could *feel* His divine presence as usual, and it was beautiful!

Cammie and her family attended mass. It seemed that the homily highlighted the fruitful life of her husband and all those who have triumphed over adversity.

Father Damian's comments brought to focus the lives of great musicians, writers and painters who have triumphed over adversity. He implied that our true blessings often appear to us in the shape of pain, losses, sufferings and disappointments. And oftentimes, beneath our adversities is a creative talent that we would not have developed had the pain not occurred. Oftentimes, creativity is born in suffering, which tells us all that suffering brings out the divine gifts God has planted within us when we use the suffering as a blessing. Suffering should be viewed as a gift from God designed to help us unlock our divine inheritance.

7

"The tragedy of life is not death, but what we let die within us."

This morning, and while meditating as usual, I was thinking about Cammie and her deceased spouse. Suddenly, a thought flashed before me. It was a philosophy my husband had given me when he was first diagnosed with multiple sclerosis, and ever since then I have embraced the wisdom because it promotes inner peace.

John said that when he was in Korea, the Chaplain told them that "The Tragedy of life is not death, but what we let die within us." He implied that we should decide to be happy and render others happy. We should proclaim our joy; love compassionately our miraculous life; and do not listen to promises. We should not wait for a better world, but be grateful for every moment of life in this world. The Chaplain told them to switch on the positive buttons in themselves, those marked optimism, serenity, confidence, positive thinking. He advised them to love, pray and thank God every day; to meditate, smile, laugh, whistle, sing, dance; to look with fascination at everything, and to fill their lungs and hearts with liberty. He counseled them to be themselves fully and immensely, to act like kings until death; to feel God in their bodies, minds, hearts and souls, and to be convinced of eternal life.

It is no wonder my husband wanted me to send his story to Mrs. Susan Ward, the public relations director of Miami's VA Medical Center, when she was collecting stories from the vets for *Chicken Soup for the Veteran's Soul.* It would have fitted in perfectly with the kinds of stories I was reading to him, but it needed to be quickly shortened because the deadline was only two hours away. Inasmuch as my higher self did not immediately suggest it because of the stress involved, none of the spirits rushed in to suggest it either.

Just now, my higher self is telling me to send in John's story because he wants to share the terrific experience that, in spite of MS, molded his character, enabling him to dedicate his life in the vocation of touching lives and lifting spirits.

Perhaps I am locked into gratitude journal writing this morning because John has pneumonia and I am writing through the pain, as usual, for therapeutic reasons. He has often said "always remember that things could be worse," and that "We should be thankful for all the things that didn't happen to us that could have happened to us."

The stories about our disabled veterans help us family caregivers to better understand what our loved ones have endured to protect our country, even at the risk of losing their own health and lives. Their courage must always be respected.

It was in the Korean War where John, along with millions of combat veterans, lost his health.

Chicken Soup for the Veteran's Soul has really stirred the hearts of many family caregivers who care for their disabled loved ones who are veterans and who share so many human experiences with us caregiving wives. Our veterans teach us that the military service, too, touches lives and lifts spirits in spite of the perils of bloody war, debilitating illnesses and disabilities.

And in the words of the song by Frank Mason North entitled *Where Cross the Crowded Ways of Life*, we learn from a spiritual viewpoint that war can indeed be an act of selfish strife. War teaches us that the Creator is speaking to us through human experiences, and many of us followers are listening attentively to Him. *Above the noise of selfish strife, we hear thy voice , O Son of Man. ...from paths where hide the lures of greed, we catch a vision of thy tears.*

FOCUS TWO: VISION

And the wondering traveler asked, "Kind Master, why are there so many disabled veterans in this world?" The Master replied, "They are here to teach you, my child, to be a candlelight for the world."

Yesterday morning, when I returned from mass and read to my husband stories from *Chicken Soup for the Veteran's Soul*, his eyes lit up and he was overwhelmed by emotion, especially when I read the story "Christmas in Korea." For some reason he felt very sure that the author's name, Larry Ebsch, was the name of the same United States army medic and kind soldier who rescued him when he was thrown from a speeding rickshaw at Camp Schimm Honshu, Japan.

The miracle that John was found will always make me grateful to those who touch lives and lift spirits. So deeply touched by his enthusiastic response, I decided to shortened his story from *Mysterious Stranger Aboard* and have the *Chicken Soup for the Soul* enterprise add it to their collection. Inasmuch as the book was written in our alternating voices, John's Turn and Alice's Turn, I will project John's turn and his account of his Korean War experiences.

Indeed, we caregiving spouses of disabled veterans share a common bond. We love to talk about our husbands' war experiences, and we talk about them with excitement as though we, too, were on the scene. We feel very proud of them and have learned from their experiences the joy of being kind and compassionate, grateful, humble and most of all spiritually supportive. Their disabilities have taught us the wisdom of love. Through them, we catch the vision of being one in the spirit of brotherly love.

Chicken Soup for the Veteran's Soul is so interesting and

entertaining, it awakens us again to how our veterans throughout America have touched our lives and lifted our spirits, making it possible for us to live in a time and place of freedom.

John admitted that the time he spent in service was one of the best experiences of his life, even though his MS did surface during that time. As his caregiving spouse, I now feel the responsibility to accede to his request and share his story, which he so enthusiastically wrote long before Hurricane Andrew blew away his prolific world.

An Excerpt from *MYSTERIOUS STRANGER ABOARD* *1951-1953*

Men are so accustomed to maintaining the external order of life by violence that they cannot conceive of life being possible without violence. (Anonymous)

John's Turn

It was one of the bloodiest wars in history, a violent, seesaw battle which claimed 54,256 American lives in three years of fighting, and 103,000 wounded. More than a million civilian men, women and children of Korea were killed, and several million made homeless. It was the Korean War—-a war in which my first classic symptoms of multiple sclerosis manifested, though the diagnosis was unknown to me at that time, while I was on duty.

The Korean War began at 4 a.m. Korean time, Sunday, June 25, 1950. More than 110,000 North Korean soldiers supported by 126 tanks and 1,400 artillery pieces rolled over the 38th Parallel, which divided North and South Korea.

It had been a period of high tension in the Cold War, and American diplomats were expecting a test somewhere. They were caught by surprise, however, when the test came in Korea.

Within two days, the American-backed government of South Korea fled the capital of Seoul and pleaded for American aid. In Washington, all agreed that South Korea had no strategic importance for the United States, but other key issues were raised by the invasion.

President Harry Truman quickly sponsored a United Nations resolution calling for armed assistance for South Korea. On June 26, he ordered U. S. ships and airplanes into combat. Four days later, ground troops were committed.

During a press conference that week, Truman said, "We are not at war." He called the effort a "police action."

"Try using that phrase with the 103,000 Americans wounded in Korea," wrote columnist Charles Whited in *The Miami Herald* forty years later. He, too, had served in that war. Or try using that phrase with the hundreds of thousands of others, like myself, who also fought there, or with our relatives such as my parents and my caregiving wife, Alice, who have had life changing experiences as a result of what happened there.

Yes, the Korean War claimed 54,246 American lives during three years and one month of conflict, compared to the Vietnam War which, in 12 years, claimed more than 58,135 American lives.

I was called to serve in the Korean War in February of 1951, hardly prepared for the ferocity of fighting or for the climatic conditions. In winter, arctic cold; summer, searing heat. I felt tingling sensations then on the left side of my body but ignored them.

During the early months, our units were under-trained, poorly equipped and below proper troop strengths—-a result of rapid demobilization after World War II.

Yes, it was cold. Thirty-five, sometimes forty below zero, and the mountains offered no shelter. We did not have the proper equipment for an arctic environment. Frostbite? Yes, my feet and both my hands. In combat, we took very heavy casualties from North Korean Communists and Communist Chinese.

Death was everywhere and it seemed such a saddening waste. I began to wonder what meaning does life have that death doesn't destroy, and what has religion taught us? "To love God and to love thy neighbor as thyself," I seemed to hear my grandmother whisper in the cold, blowing winds where lifeless bodies of my brothers laid. I fell to my knees in prayer, searching for answers to this bloodcurdling experience that made life a living hell.

The answers sneaked in under the umbrella of MS... More Suffering. Another form of bloody war—a hidden agenda—destined to destroy one's life.

It was following an accident in Japan when I first experienced definite symptoms of what was twenty years later diagnosed as multiple sclerosis, sometimes called MS. Multiple sclerosis is a chronic disease of the central nervous system that robs motor skills. Yes, it was another kind of destructive war inching in to destroy my life.

On the night of March 4, 1954, my army friend, Charlie, and I were enroute back to camp when, suddenly he lost control of the speeding rickshaw.

"Oh-o-o-o!" I screamed as we were thrown from the vehicle.

The silence smelled of death as darkness blanketed the skies. I lay there in an eerie stillness, a crawling sensation trickling down my face. Panic gripped me.

"Charlie!" I called to my friend, only to have my call returned by a distant echo.

Slowly, I raised my hands to touch the trickling. Its texture and odor made me aware that it was blood.

Dear God, don't let me die, I pleaded in silence, fighting to keep my eyes open and to remain conscious. Stinging sensations seized my left side which were later replaced by a feeling of numbness.

A million thoughts raced through my mind as I tried to get to my feet. Every effort failed. I lay there in the darkness praying to live, frightfully realizing how precious life is. Mom, Dad, Grandma, Grandpa, Uncle Horse, Uncle Jake, beautiful Cincinnati, Ohio...would I see them all again? " Dear God, please, I don't want to die!"

It seemed I heard my mother's prayer, her voice tender and reassuring singing, "God will take care of you." Suddenly, a feeling of calmness stilled my fear. I relaxed and continued praying, thanking God for 22 years of precious life, and for my lovely family, friends, army buddies and the world... all His holy creation.

My last memory while lying there was the wailing sound of sirens, growing. My next recollection was being awakened by the chief of surgery. I had been in the hospital three days, totally unaware of what took place during that period. Later that week, I learned that the orthopedic clinical record and surgical consultation revealed that I had severe abrasions on the right forehead and cheek; severe contusion on the upper lip and cheek and a fractured right parietal bone. The doctor recommended that I remain in the hospital three weeks from the date of injury for necessary treatment.

Following a series of x-rays and treatments, I was discharged to full duty. The army chaplain informed me that my good buddy, Charlie, was killed in the accident. I wept. Later I learned that my mother had seen the accident in a dream even before it actually happened. She had wept so hysterically that the entire church was praying for her, that she might maintain sanity.

Although my life was spared following the accident, my good health wasn't. My ability to see clearly was now a problem because I was experiencing blurred vision, blind spots and a decrease in brightness. Following an examination, prescription glasses were ordered. The problems persisted sporadically along with tingling sensations in my left arm and leg, especially while in combat; and urinary frequency and urgency. But I attributed these heath problems to excessive stress, weather conditions and the war. Thus, I continued with my duties, too afraid to envision this situation as a fatal illness. I recall that during this period, I was demoted from sergeant to corporal because my physical condition interfered with my ability to satisfactorily perform, even though I was putting forth my best efforts as a soldier to be strong, proud and courageous, even in combat.

Yes, we Americans fought a tension-filled war in the icy mountains against suicidal swarms of North Korean Communist and Chinese. But there was one blessing for which I was grateful. The army turned boys into men. Being in the army taught me the basic psychology of overcoming fear and gaining confidence in every phase of life. Fighting in the Korean War, there was no escape for me from this process. Here, I learned that every step in the conquest of fear requires an act of will.

On February 7, 1953, I was honorably discharged, and was extremely proud that I had been called to serve my country.

Having served in this oftentimes-forgotten war, I knew that my life, physically, spiritually and mentally, would never be the same.

Twenty years after being discharged, I was officially diagnosed with MS although the symptoms were present following the rickshaw accident, and had been sporadically flaring up, slowly becoming worse and worse each year before being officially diagnosed. Research has found that even though one might be carrying the MS gene, it usually flares up as a result of a serious fall or accident.

Utilizing the wisdom gained from being in the army, I completed my college education, earned the doctorate degree in education, and devoted my life to continue serving humanity, in spite of my debilitating disease. On the journey, I learned from both the army and my illness that greater than life is our personal relationship with God, who commands us to love one another and who awakens us to transcendent wisdom and universal compassion.

FOCUS THREE: THE ENLIGHTENMENT

Do not consider painful what is good for you.
—Euripides

Today, I can readily recall the kindness and concern of others who helped us open the doors to enlightenment when John's illness was finally diagnosed as multiple sclerosis. With the help of counselors, whose mission is to touch lives and lift spirits, we were able to deal with life's negative experiences by shifting gears through poetry therapy. How well I remember the thoughts and feelings that shaped our world when we let our emotions speak through the pain that led to the spiritual path of enlightenment .

The following poems were written in 1978 when John and I were enrolled in a poetry class at the University of Miami.

SHIFTING GEARS

At first the sun stood still
When MS eased into a chapter
of our anchored life
and stood with clenched fists
to claim remaining
pages of a volume
yet unwritten.

We paused, but for a moment
to gather ourselves
and document its
untimely entrance
as we, in silence, wept

mid dismal clouds
of mirrored hopelessness.

But then, instead, each day embraced
a strange new spiritual growth.
With sharing wings,
a glowing light of human understanding
illuminated each new page
as we danced through added chapters
in shifted gears.

And we, in writing,
continue in richness
of soul that MS brings.....enlightened.
For love is its own reason.

DETOURING

My mind is a library
shelved with volumed documents
of million yesterworlds.
It steers me through new day
in choice titles.
And carves my universe.

In passing through,
I sometimes stop to sweep away cobwebs
from outdated stacks
as I frustrate through new data in logic search. I detour,
and move through volume fiction escapades
to fantasize creations where I control ALL MINDS!
I search for inner peace.

Through chapter-islands of great ancient classics
biographies, music, art...
columned in each school,
my joy emotions wing in selected taste...
some live; some die into the nothingness
strangled by green forest's twisted vines,
And blocked sun bridges.

Oftentimes
mysteries beckon
swinging me through question-tunnels where I,
on hypotheses, dine. I overeat space in
my too seriousness, and escape through pages of
litter in wide-eyed consciousness.
I feel guilt-bored.

Bible-stares pierce
on turbulent mind, sprinkling
wrathful blood on my childish guilt.
I am frustrated. I hate the god of my
ignorance. The "I-me-it" illusion.
At detour, I set course to destroy him
by rising to higher consciousness in intellectual's
cosmic imagery.

I image,
and linger on shelves stocked
with philosophy old. And pause
to brush away accumulated dust. Through
flipped pages, my vision grabs spirit-rocks
and pocket them.
Some are real. Some simulated.
Molding me.

Starved and athirst,
I detour to drink from
creation's selected volumes,
and slowly restock my mind's library
with gift-blessings of inherited divinity.
'Twas when I find that LOVE is always
the only and perfect answer.
I am the joy of enlightened life!

DRY NOT MY TEARS

(For John, on the sudden death of his beloved mother)

Dry not my tears
but let me dwell within
the dismal walls of pensive grief
and listen to my inner soul
pound out its rage
in choked-full utterance.
Through grief we find our strengths.

For though within "Celestial" scenes
of yonder world
sightless to mortal mind,
my tears bespeak the sorrow
thus embedded.
I dare now bid adieu her earthly exit.
And let my tears awaken worlds of enlightenment.

O' SILENT GRAVE

O' silent grave
O' cold and silent grave
    that bleeds my tortured soul
    to depths of endless pain
        with moans
        unuttered,
    speak gently
    to these stolid tears that have
    disrupted in their course
    my tranquil state of
    pensive equilibrium
And let me feel but spiritual awakening.
I am enlightened.

WHERE PARAGONS MEET

The purple morning
    faded into a paragon of beauty
    awakening with its cloudless layers
        creation's zealous naturemates
        from, their
    sleepless vale.

And I, adrift in the quietude
    of thought,
    breathed a "mantra"
        to give priority's depth
        to my agendaed day
    through pulse-rhythm litanies.

The apologetic jingle of a telephone
with its disruptive sonnet
snapped consciousness
into my "mantra-world"
I answered
only to be awakened once again...

But this time to a colorless morning
that faded into a paragon of horror
triggered by the tragic death
of one so loved
who taught us how to love
and feel the love.

But what is sorrow but a prelude to our happiness.
Let nature run its course.
Joy gains its glory out of sorrow,
bitter sorrow and man's loneliness.
So, let my heart embrace the sadness
then let go.

For dark and light are both alike to Him
who created joy and sadness
where paragons meet
to take us to new heights
of spiritual growth.
And thus we are enlightened.
For joy is one's brother.

"I sought my God, and He withdrew from me; I sought my soul, and it eluded me; I sought my brother, in him I found all three."

FOCUS FOUR: THE FULFILLMENT

The greatest fulfillment we can ever experience is the joy of loving God and doing His will.

Today when I visited my husband, I again read to him enjoyable stories from *Chicken Soup for the Veteran's Soul*. Veterans share a common bond of feeling love and compassion for one another. The book attests to this truth.

My husband is still confined to bed due to pneumonia, and is still being intravenously administered antibiotics.

After applauding John for being in good spirits even though he is confined to bed because of his illness, I talked about the courage he has shown throughout his life as a veteran. He has displayed a soldier's strength in spite of multiple sclerosis and its debilitating effects. His courage is typical of many of the veterans whose stories were included in *Chicken Soup for the Veteran's Soul.*

In all of the stories, we saw acts of compassion, kindness and concern. Perhaps this is what makes the experiences they describe so delightful...people doing the will of God by helping one another.

When I read "Remembrance Day" written by Christine Ann Maxwell-Osborn, John and I both had watery eyes. We were moved by the compassion displayed between a war captain and his young soldiers, who were fighting a bloody battle. In the story, the captain was haunted by the faces of the boys he had to order into battle, the ones who would never come back. In one of the battles, a young friend wanted to go into a war zone to see if his buddy was still alive and needed help. The captain knew that to let him go would mean sudden death. But the young friend was insistent. "He could be lying out there hurt. I must go find him." The pleading look in the young man's eyes touched the captain. "I am sorry, son, to let you go back here would be suicidal." Tearfully, the young man continued to plead. But the captain was adamant, ordering the young man to go back to his post. He knew that to send him into the war-torn area would be to condemn him to death. "Soldier, I'm sorry, your friend is probably dead. What purpose would it serve to let you sacrifice your life, too?"

"At least I'd know I'd tried, sir. He'd do the same thing in my shoes, I know he would."

The captain was about to order the boy back to the rank again but the impact of his words softened his heart even more. He saw himself in the young man then said, All right, soldier, you can go." The young man smiled. "Thank you, sir! God bless you, sir!" He hurried off to find his friend. Hours later, he found him, wounded and dying. The soldier held his dying friend in his arms and heard him whisper, "I knew you'd come."

Yes, the soldier found his friend who died in his arms. In his search, the soldier was critically wounded and he told his story to the captain from his hospital bed.

It is interesting how all the stories reveal the power of kindness. The series itself is an institution for learning that kindness is the art of touching lives and lifting spirits.

The key to spiritual fulfillment for modern man in this twenty-first century lies in the fullest possible development of his own humanity. Caregiving experiences have taught us that old-time practices of silent prayer and withdrawal from the world are still relevant in today's age. But even more relevant is a life of kindness. To become fully human we must be awakened through visions of enlightenment and fulfillment, and feel the love within us for one another. We must be present to our fellow man. Man will reach God only through his brother, for there he will find Christ.

Jesus of Nazareth's fully human life here on planet earth is the most perfect example of all humanity and the ideal on which we must model our lives in order to realize our awakening, vision, enlightenment and fulfillment. His life here on earth is the epitome of human kindness.

2
The Hidden Power of Human Kindness

This morning at our daily mass service, I was given a *Christian Action* newsletter that caught my attention because it contained an article about the hidden power of kindness. Coincidentally, I am writing a book entitled *Kindness is the True Religion.*

The truth is, kindness is all around us but we fail to notice it because we are too busy with our own agendas. Luckily, through gratitude journal writing, John and I have been able to see a world of kindness because gratitude journal writing is therapeutic. It helps us to *feel* the love that surrounds us in our everyday experiences.

We as humans need encouragement and oftentimes praise that gives us moral support. Kindness encompasses all the virtues of praise without its vanity. While it is true that praise may encourage pride, kindness enriches those who are kind to you.

Life teaches us that kindness is indeed the most graceful attitude you can extend toward another. A kind deed, a kind word, a kind tone of voice can touch lives and lift spirits like no other activity can.

When kindness calls for self-denial and the spirit of helping others to feel appreciated, loved and respected, the sacrifice is both noble and rewarding.

Fortunately, at the VA Medical Center, we often see this kind of love in action. The following is a poem with thoughts and feelings dictated by my husband and written into poetic verse by me inasmuch as Hurricane Andrew stilled his prolific voice. The poem emphasizes how the VA staff members, through acts of kindness, touch the lives and lift the spirits of our disabled veterans...our brothers.

WE VETERANS HAD A PICNIC
by John Johnson
(via caregiver/ghost-writer/wife, Alice)

We had a picnic yesterday and we had lots of fun!
And those who planned it
made us feel that "Vets Are Number One!"
The picnic was on April twelve at beautiful Barnes Park;
Our caring VA staff made us as happy as a lark!

They took us there on VA buses; we enjoyed the ride;
They made us all feel special as we vets rode side by side;
Kala Vidal checked off our names as we got on each bus;
She, Cynthia Braithwaite and her staff stayed busy helping us.

There are a lot of staff members whose names I do not know
Who did outstanding jobs in helping us...each was a pro!
Yes, the whole staff of workers are indeed professional;
They took us safely there and back. They are exceptional!

They pushed our wheelchairs gently
as they handled us with care;
They helped us board the buses
and they carefully drove us there;
They treated us like war heroes and we truly felt love;

This type of kindness and concern we never grow tired of.
When we arrived at Barnes Park our food awaited us;
"Yum-yum! we said while being wheeled
from our smooth riding bus;
The music was fantastic; juicy hot dogs, burgers, too!
We gobbled down delicious foods
and thanked the cooking crew.

We had a good time singing, both in and out of tune;
We "shook-a-leg," patted our feet. I danced with my balloon;
Vera and her Punorno and my Alice clapped along
As the musicians played the "You are My Sunshine" song.

We thank the nursing/caring staff for a delightful day!
They made us vets feel special in a very special way,
They touched our lives, lifted our spirits,
made us Number One;
The picnic was fantastic! Oh, boy, did we have fun!

Epilogue

The pilgrim stranger, through family caregiving experiences, had learned that when we devote ourselves to the joy of touching lives and lifting spirits, we are showing the world that kindness is, indeed, the true religion because kindness purifies, glorifies and ennobles all that it touches and lifts.

The pilgrim stranger learned from her disabled brother that gratitude journaling enables us to follow the path that leads to fulfillment. Journaling gives us the joy of talking to one's higher self while at the same time meditating silently and seeing the spiritual message each personal experience entails.

Meditating on what the messages of life had taught, the

traveler looked within and saw the continuity of the spiritual keys for avoiding caregiver-burnout and promoting inner peace. As a spiritual guide to contentment, joy and fulfillment, the basic message taught her to trust life and it would teach her. Focusing the light within, she saw the vision of life's caregiving wisdom and read the message to light her candle and share it with the world.

Trust Life and it Will Teach You

Life teaches us through human experiences the joy of truly being kind, and that many devout people are actually unkind but are unaware of it. Oftentimes, we have to say: *Father, forgive them for they know not what they do.* We have seen that in many instances people may be charitable, merciful, self-sacrificing, polite, compassionate, understanding, but are not kind. They do not feel the love within themselves. Kindness is, indeed, the main purpose of God's presence in the world and in our hearts.

"Be ye kind to one another" is what the kind Master commanded. And when we truly love God and obey His will by being kind to one another, we are at our highest peak of happiness, for we *feel the love* within us. It is indeed "the high" we all seek; it is the epitome of touching lives and lifting spirits...a pathway to God through our daily relationships with our neighbors.

The power of touching lives and lifting spirits through acts of kindness is not in what it does for us, but in where it leads us: immediately to the heart of all humanity and therefore to our Eternal God who dwells within us all. Touching lives and lifting spirits can be seen as an anticipation of the ultimate: the presence of heaven in our earthly life, the poetic sounds of gratitude.

Spiritual Key # 5

Poetry Therapy and the Family Caregiver

Gratitude journal writing is a form of poetry therapy that reaffirms the soul. It is the memory of the heart.

FOREWORD

Poetry is a Candlelight of Thoughts and Feelings

Prelude

Feeling the need to view the world of caregiving as a song, the pilgrim stranger asked, "Kind master, how can my disabled brother teach me to hear music that speaks of the deeds of kindness and expressions of gratitude in my world of caregiving?"

"My dear child," the kind Master whispered, "you must listen quietly to the world of your disabled brother and your caregiving. Then meditating by candlelight, use your spiritual keys and unlock the kindness that every experience portrays, and let the poetry within you write its message."

Of Thoughts and Feelings

Poetry is a way of finding God within oneself...in the kind, creative, fulfilled individual.

My husband's first book of poetry, written during the early stages of his MS diagnosis, was entitled *Of Thoughts and Feelings*. It is the book that gave him wisdom to trust life because life is the greatest teacher. It taught him by living examples that God is life. When my husband was awakened by this powerful message, he lit his candle and shared the light with me.

Using the flame from his candle, I took it and, running like hell from a world of caregiver-burnout, wrote my first book of poetry entitled *Poetry Therapy: How to Feel Good About Yourself.* The University of Miami Department of Psychiatry chairman, Dr. Sussex, wrote the foreword for my book of poetry. The following is an excerpt from his message:

All of us see the world in two ways. First in ways that are generally shared by most others in the culture, and second, in many ways that are unique to us as individuals—-ways of interpreting things and explaining things to ourselves that have grown out of our own highly personal and frequently very private experiences. When one is afflicted by clinical depressions, it is common to find these two ways of looking at the world in conflict with each other, and these conflicting views lead to perplexity, anxiety and sometimes panic. It may feel as if we have lost all means of understanding other people and that they no longer understand us. Communication becomes extremely difficult, and we feel (and are regarded by those around us) alienated. It isn't accidental that psychiatrists were once called 'alienists." And alienated people are almost always miserable people. Other people do not feel good about them and they do not feel good about themselves.

Poets, like other artists, write not only for the usual events common to our everyday life, nor of the exotic aspects of other cultures—although these may be the easels on which their poetry is sketched out. They write also from those feelings and fantasies that are common to all of us but which may not be buried deeply in our unconscious minds, too deeply to be recognized easily or to be elicited in ordinary conversation. The "free association" of psychoanalysis is one way of helping these submerged thoughts and feelings come into consciousness. ...The important thing is that the patient is likely to find in the poetry meanings that are significant for himself/ herself. The therapist can help the patient weave these new thoughts and feelings into a new self image. ...Feeling good about the self, as the title of this inspiring volume so aptly implies, is necessary for good physical, mental and spiritual health and happiness.

Fortunately, my psychologist was able to guide me in using my therapy to write through the stages of depression and unmask my true self-image. With this new image, I was able to feel good about myself, the world of caregiving and the world around me.

VISION ONE
Life is a Poetic Song of Candlelights

O Lord I will give thanks to you forever.
— Psalm 30:12

The Beauty of Gratitude Journaling and Poetic Verse

When gratitude journal writing is composed in poetic verse, it expresses our most intimate feelings of love, gratitude, friendship, grief, memory, faith and inspiration. It captures in a few words the thoughts, feelings and emotions that reach to the heart of human experience, sending a light into the universal truth that unites all of us...love. It unites the patient with the caregiver; it unites the reader with the world and becomes a poetic song of candlelights..

Gratitude journal writing in poetic verse is holistic medicine that teaches us through everyday caregiving experiences that the body is the servant of the mind. The body obeys the operations of the mind. This mind/body medicine helps us to see through personal experiences that disease and health, like circumstances, are rooted in thoughts, feelings and emotions.

When we entertain an attitude of ingratitude or negative thoughts, the body sinks rapidly into disease and decay. On the other hand, when we entertain an attitude of gratitude or positive thoughts, the body becomes clothed in beauty.

Gratitude journal writing is a form of poetry therapy that can have a positive effect on our health. There is no physician like poetry therapy for dissipating the ills of the body, mind and spirit. There is no comforter to compare with poetry therapy for dispersing the shadows of grief and sorrow.

Poetry therapy through gratitude journal writing is an activity that can help us come out of our self-made prison holes or thoughts of ill will, cynicism, suspicion and fear. It helps us to think well of all people, to be cheerful with all, to patiently learn to find the good in all and to feel the beauty within ourselves.

Poetry Therapy is Mind/Body Medicine

Poetry therapy is holistic healing...mind/body medicine, for the caregiver and the patient, in that it gives them a prescription expressing their thoughts and feelings in healthy avenues of the soul. It is one of the natural devices which the caregiver and patient can engage in to cope with the inevitable crises of living. The caregiver becomes both the ministering 'therapist" and the comforted "patient" while writing for the care recipient.

This section on poetry therapy is the result of John's and my meditations and experiences that promote our spiritual growth and well being. It is designed to help motivate caregivers and their patients to discover the truth that life is a poem of unending gratitude, humility and praise. Just "to be" is a blessing; Just "to live" is indeed holy.

In this volume are poems of gratitude that project the human experiences of kindness, faith, compassion, sacrifice, truth, romance, marriage, family; poems that tell a story, reaffirm the soul, touch lives and lift spirits.

It is patterned to help the caregiver and recipient appreciate the people surrounding them in their visions, thoughts, feelings and emotions; and to express their feelings of gratitude. Like gratitude journal writing, poetry therapy awakens an understanding of the inner self and helps us to know our own inner greatness and prosperity when we learn to say "thank you."

The more we engage in the silence of poetic gratitude journal writing and meditation, the more we unlock our own world of abundant happiness.

The poems in this chapter celebrate the joy of loving, respecting and appreciating staff and patients in the Veterans Administration Medical Center and nursing home who play major roles in touching lives and lifting spirits to promote a spiritual climate of joy and inner peace. The experiences made music in our world of caregiving and they became a poetic song of candlelights.

2

Christ peace must reign in your heart, since as members of one body, you have been called to that peace.
Dedicate yourself to thankfulness.
—Colossians 3:15

Poetry Therapy and the Human Spirit

On life's spiritual journey, caregiving experiences have taught us that gratitude journal writing while caring for a loved one is a mysterious awakening that taps the creative spirit within us and our care recipient, exploring wonders. It is the human spirit of self-discovery through self-expression. It is poetry therapy for the mind, body and soul.

We all have thoughts, feelings and emotions that can be creatively expressed through *poetry therapy.* One of the joyful ways of being a compassionate caregiver is to work cooperatively with our care patient in writing various styles of poetry and/or prose expressing gratitude for the purpose of reciprocally touching lives and lifting spirits.

What is life but a song...a song of human experiences that come from the depths of the soul. What is a song but beautiful poetry that speaks from a grateful heart.

Poetry is used in gratitude journal writing to share deep feelings of the human mind as we paint our worlds with positive words of gratitude. In so doing, we bring about inner discipline within ourselves while cultivating spiritual thoughts and feelings in reference to our daily experiences.

What is gratitude journal writing but a poem that opens us to moments of grace, quietness, solitude. Gratitude journal writing is a myriad of poems that enable us to see and feel all the wonders and kindnesses in our world of people around us who are forever touching lives and lifting spirits.

Reasons for Writing "Poetry Therapy and the Caregiver"

When the murderous windstorms of Hurricane Andrew blew my totally disabled husband, John, into Miami's Veterans Administration Medical Center Nursing Home in 1992, I was terrified with fear. I had heard so many negative reports about nursing home neglect that my frightened mind would not let me think otherwise. I did not realize at that time that our lives would become whatever our thoughts are, and I was burdened with suspicion, ingratitude and fear.

Quickly, I realized that the effects of this ugly, negative attitude was evolving into feelings of chronic depression. I rushed to my analyst, Dr. Kensinger, for suggestions in helping me cope with the excessive stress. I knew from previous counseling that feelings of ugliness lower our vitality and disturb our digestion and our nerves, creating caregiver-burnout, whereas an attitude of inner beauty is the promise of joy and inner peace.

My analyst wisely suggested that I use my poetry therapy to heal my troubled thoughts and feelings; and to remember that human beings can alter their lives by alternating their attitudes of mind.

"Alice, you can think your way out of any difficult situation or problem regarding your fears of nursing homes," he had counseled. Then gesturing with opened palms, he smiled and gently continued, "At the VA hospital nursing home, your husband will be receiving 24-hour professional care. Alice, you're not a medical specialist; and you're not equipped with the resources to give him this kind of professional help. You should feel grateful for professional help."

I wanted to tell him that I was a caregiver-burnout specialist, running like hell trying to combat the stress. After all, John and I were in the process of completing our emotion-packed autobiography, *Mysterious Stranger Aboard.*

In my fight to "Shun not the struggle, face it; 'tis God's gift...be strong" I needed a miracle to help modify my already overloaded attitude of ungratefulness regarding the nursing home odyssey. To John and me, the thought of placing him in a nursing facility was akin to our paranoid feelings of Hurricane Andrew, the destructive windstorm that had blown him to VA's nursing home.

3

Gratitude From the Heart

After lighting my candle and meditating for hours about the nursing home, my feelings of gratitude emerged, then flowed into a medley of poems. I shared my feelings with John. He loved the idea and suggested that we write our thoughts and feelings. Immediately and with a passion, he and I entered our world of poetry and began writing non-stop. The experience was, indeed, a spiritual key that saved me from the wrath of caregiver-burnout and promoted our inner peace.

This spiritual key of poetry therapy was written to highlight the good deeds of kind people at the nursing facility who are touching lives and lifting spirits. It is a poetic expression of sincere gratitude compiled from experiences recorded in our gratitude journals. Although the contents of the poems basically portray my husband's gratitude, as he speaks not only for himself but oftentimes for his fellow residents, I am the caregiving ghostwriter. As a family caregiver, I feel that it is my responsibility to give my husband moral support by encouraging him to express his gratitude and to *feel* the love. In so doing, I am also helping myself to *feel* the love and gratitude within. John and I have been healing each other through gratitude journal writing and poetry therapy, using them as spiritual keys.

Poetry Therapy and the Caregiver is designed to show how the family caregiver can help his/her disabled loved one cooperatively release those inner thoughts and feelings of love and joy. It is a poetic method of lighting candles within one's world and letting them shine throughout the world.

A Nursing Staff of Angels as Candlelights

When we accept the truism that all creation is holy, hospitals and nursing homes become great institutions of learning, not only for the staff but also for the patients and family caregivers who see creation's kingdom in action...from sanitary engineers to the most serious medical professionals.

Family caregiving with gratitude journaling about nursing homes enables the insightful caregiver to see the depths of man's interconnectedness, interrelatedness and interdependence in the kingdom of products and services. Caregiving awakens the caregiver to the knowledge that the joy in labor is a direct line of creation, from God, through man, to mankind. And that we as laborers must be humble before God, yet great in Him as we perform our missions in the spirit of love and kindness.

As we listen poetically to the many choirs of the universe harmonizing, we see the beauty and intelligence of creation;

we feel the joy of realizing that we multi-cultural, multi-ethnic, multi-gifted humans are all co-creators with God; and we see a nursing staff of candlelights, transforming the world, one kind deed at a time.

VISION TWO
Candlelights of Gratitude and Kindness

By VA patient John Johnson
and ghostwriter/caregiver/wife Alice

The test of a people is how it behaves toward the old and disabled. It is easy to love children...but affection and care for the old, the incurable, the helpless are the true gold mines of a culture. —Rabbi Abraham Joshua Heschel

A PRELUDE IN GRATITUDE TO THE VA MEDICAL CENTER AND NURSING HOME

To VA, our poetic half
Who likes to make us think and laugh
Who gives our thoughts poetic verse
To put our illness in reverse.

By using Macintosh software
And VA's staff Nursing Home care
We write journals of gratitude
our thoughts and feelings all include...

Experiences that bring us joy,
Transcendent wisdom that employ
Symbols of love that have renewed
Our attitude of gratitude.

ABOUT US VETERANS

Well, here we are at VA, a hospital for us vets
And as disabled veterans we never shall forget
We fought in our country's wars
In case you're wondering "what for?"
We're loyal, brave...Oh, yes, we are!
And we have no regrets.

We're war veterans from everywhere,
Our bodies bear the scars
Some of us fought in Vietnam
And some in the World Wars
Some of us fought in South Korea
Where freezing cold knew no degrees
And scorching heat was fiery.
'Twas for a noble cause.

We love the way America
Cares for its DAVs
With caring social workers
We're given dignities.
The doctors work within a team
Some are terrific, some between
But good teamwork is always seen
Indeed, professionally.

The nurses are like angels
At least, most of them are
Some have the patience of a saint
But we're not saints by far
Our illnesses are so diverse
We're thankful for each caring nurse

So let's applaud VA in verse
We DVAs of WAR.

WE OWE SO MANY 'THANK YOU' HUGS TO VA's PERSONNEL

We owe so many "Thank You" hugs
To VA's personnel
We know them by their beautiful smiles,
But their names we misspell.

VA's admission directors
Always greet us with their smiles
Convey to us that VA always
Goes those extra miles.

Because of this endeavor, we would
Like to say "Thank You!"
You make us all feel welcome
Patients, friends and families, too.

We thank our VA doctors for
Their medical advice
And for professional services
That keep us well and wise.

We thank caregiving nurses
For tender, loving care
We see the genius of their works
In action everywhere.

We thank our patient nursing aids
Who help us help ourselves
when our hands are far too weak
Our bodies in despair.

We thank the cleaning/cooking staff
And those who fix wheelchairs;
Thanks to the many caregivers
Their work's beyond compare.

There's so much love at VA
And we see it everyday
We thank Administration for
This wonderful display.

Thus, in poetic verse with
my dear friends and family, too
We happy voices of VA
Would like to say "THANK YOU!"

IN GRATITUDE TO THE NURSING HOME

We humans are a gift to one another
We humans love to love and help each other
We humans love to say
"And how are you today?"
In our VA sister/brother way.

We learn through deeds the true wisdom of love
That wings its flight and makes us turtle doves
It is the master-mind

That makes us culture blind
We humans are a gift to humankind.

It is our task to sell the world on love
It's a philosophy we've all thought of
Love is a healthy diet
That gives our goal sunlight
and paints our whole world beautiful, thereof.

VA taught us of healing and the mind
We know that happy thoughts can be defined
As thoughts that say "VA,
We love your 'caring' way
We thank you; you're a blessing to mankind."

And here at VA we engage in games
In which our teachers know us all by name
"We feel valued, of course,
Because staff members know
The names of all us patients," I exclaimed.

The art of being grateful can be learned
And learned we have at VA where concern
Has always been a craft
Of VA's nursing staff
We've learned to say "I Thank You!" in return.

Here at VA we've learned what health care is
When doctors/nurses come around to quiz
They ask, "How do you feel?"
I say, "Tip-Top," for real
"Your mind and body health care is a whiz."

And with Administration's welcome smile
We catch the spirit which is kind, gentle;
We thank them for their views
For leadership they use
To teach us VA patients VA style.

FROM THE HEART TO VA NURSING HOME -2

Thank you so much for being you
You are the ideal staff;
Sometimes when we would like to cry
You often make us laugh.

We love the way you care for us
With kindness and concern;
We don't always say "Thank you, friend."
'Tis something we must learn.

We'd love to write each of your names
But we cannot because
We have been told by a kind nurse
That you've an ethical code.

"A code of ethics?" we did ask
When we requested your names.
Such modesty, humility,
Your love's a burning flame!"

Yes, we're the vets of many wars,
Disabled in the flesh
You help our spirits stay alive
With energy afresh.

We feel so special in wheelchairs,
Our beds, or with our canes;
You make us feel like heroes
And like heroes we'll remain

So, thanks to every one of you
For tender, loving care;
And we disabled vets thank God
For you in our prayers.

COUNSELOR MADELINE

In sessions with our counselor, Madeline
We have the joy of looking deep within
Our thoughts and feelings mainly we express
Experiences of contentment and distress.
Our thoughts and feelings surface and alight
The memories of things both wrong and right.

With her we feel relaxed and share our thoughts
We empty ourselves of things that thwart
The healing that our minds and bodies need
To help us all feel comfortable, indeed.

She helps us solve those problems that bring pain
Her counseling makes us feel good again.

One day she met with my Alice and me
In Madeline's atmosphere we both felt free.
And this feeling of freedom was the kind
That eased into the cobwebs of our mind.

We emptied our minds of hidden guilt
Lodged in the cobwebs that our fears had built
As a caregiver Alice felt she'd failed
Then tried to blame herself for being ill.

"No, no! That's not your fault," Madeline advised
Then gently counseled us and analyzed
How Al must rid herself of these guilt-thoughts,
Her insight was the wisdom Al had sought.

Madeline's soft spoken voice offered advice
To which we both adhered. It sounded wise.
We sealed it with joined hands as we all prayed
Repeating healing phrases Madeline said.

We were advised to keep on writing plays,
And musicals and poems...they're therapies.
And now we write of our experiences here
We thank Administration's counseling care.

We thought our writing days were over until
Our counselor, Madeline, and her boss instilled
In us the joy of being free from guilt
While having our spirit, home and life rebuilt.

Now, when my Alice visits here with me
We both go on a therapy writing spree.
We love the conversations with each friend
They're nature's masterpiece, they are godsend.

We highlight all the love in action here
That makes us all delightfully aware

That our Miami VA's number one
And counselor Madeline, ...a phenomenon!

IN TRIBUTE TO MIAMI'S VA

Let the peace of Christ control your hearts, the peace into which you were also called in one body. And be thankful.

VA hospital, we applaud
And hold you dearly to our heart
As we salute your care.
Through summer, winter, spring and fall
You are a blessing to us all
And your response to our call
Is like an answered prayer.

We shall forever sing your praise
And thank you for this lovely place
Which we all love so dear.
Yes, we war veterans of this land
We patients, families...hand-in-hand
Commend you for this wonderland
Of tender, loving care.

Your programs are a master-key
And your staff, the epitome
Of kindness and concern.
We praise the guidance that you give
To help us in our fight to live
Your service is indicative
Of tributes you have earned.

VA hospital, we thank you
For all the wonders that you do
To give us sunny days.
And in your huge circle of care
You drew us in from everywhere
Our multi-culturalness we share
We gladly give you praise.

IN GRATITUDE TO CYNTHIA FINNEY AND VA'S CITY OF ANGELS

(Social Worker, Veterans Administration Medical Center)

Our Cynthia,
A symbol of love,
in whom love finds expression
through kindness and concern,
is a portrait of eternal beauty.

When Hurricane Andrew blew away our home
that historic August 24, 1992
and left my Alice, me and my MS
locked in its terror,

my VA social worker, Cynthia,
caring for the caregiver amid
the calm and the strife
came to our rescue with her majestic
VA rescue team of angels.

I, in my world of physical disability,
watched with heartfelt gratitude and tears
as VA's vessels of love hurried me into the caring arms

of Hollywood's Washington Manor Nursing Home...
and later, closer, into Love's "Circle of Care"
at Kendall's Heartland Nursing Home;
and finally into The VA Medical Center...a learning institution
    of God's love and service in action
        Which I call "The City of Angels."
Overwhelmed
    with gratitude, joy and
        enlightenment;
From this feeling was born
    our unending world of gratitude journal writing
where we learned through daily experiences the joy of our
    spiritual interdependence
        spiritual interconnectedness
            spiritual interrelatedness
as humans!

This caregiving mystery of
    VA's love and service in action
        chronicles that love is
            the greatest creation of life.

For these spiritual awakenings and symbols of love in action,
    we are grateful!

VISION THREE
Candlelights for the World of Courage Amid Adversities

My Mysterious Stranger, Multiple Sclerosis

Mysterious Stranger does intrude
To rain on my parade
And oftentimes he's very rude
To my kind nursing aide.
I say to him, "MS, be nice."
He says to me, "Damn your advice;
I'll box your ears, punch out your eyes
This is my masquerade!"

He makes me angry and confused
And oftentimes afraid
To shower in my birthday nude
Before my nursing aide.
Sometimes the water is too cold
Which makes my MS very bold
He doesn't do as he is told
And we all feel dismayed.

Even when I'm being dressed for bed
Mysterious Stranger pouts
Sometimes he uses ugly words
That curse the nurse aides out.
He said, "Some nurse aides are too rough!
I'm getting tired of this darn stuff!
My flesh is tender, it's not tuff,
"specially my water-spout!"

I'm glad the nurses understand
This puzzling charade
And those who lend a helping-hand
Deserve an accolade.
This MS personality
Will make you feel that it is me
But 'tis the stranger as you see
That's causing this blockade.

I'm thankful for my MS friend
He taught me how to love
His teachings seem to never end
With wisdom from above.
I've learned the joy of loving life
Especially my caregiving wife
We're vessels in the calm and strife
She is my turtle dove.

MS has taught us how to write
And writing gives us joy;
MS has taught us how to fight
The pain when fears annoy.
We write journals of gratitude
Of thoughts and feelings that include
Our thankfulness for spiritual food
His lessons, we enjoy.

We thank MS for teaching us
The joy of saying "Thanks,"
For "thank-you" is a stimulus
That certainly outranks
The comments that we fail to make
For blessings we so often take

But this bad habit we can break
With MS' joyful "Thanks!"

(The following is my revised version
of a poem written by an unknown author)

GRIEF IS..

Grief is a tiring journey
One travels all alone
Upon a train of sorrow
To stations that are unknown.

The painful desolation
Bruises mind, body and soul
You feel fear and rejection
With emotions uncontrolled.

Grief is a swirling maelstrom
A vortex of fear and loss
Abandonment, with guilt and shame
And sanity at great cost.

Grief is the bridge to acceptance
That spans troubled waters deep
Peace, healing and forgiveness
Are the bounties that we reap.

Grief is a hidden message
Of blessings just for you
Though spiritual growth is painful
God's love will bring you through.

IN TRIBUTE TO GANDHI AND KING

Let us applaud Gandhi and his disciple
In their courageous nonviolent pursuit
Both men are legends, they both carved a pathway
And for their ardent work we pay tribute.

They walked with God through dangerous assignments
And followed Him with dignity and pride;
He gave them strength to love in spite of torments
Which they encountered in their freedom stride.

They led a campaign of passive resistance
To both the British and American rule;
They sought reform and it was through persistence
That they both won in spite of ridicule.

They sought political and social reform,
And economic reform peacefully.
They led with love, for love can truly transform;
They knew with love we'd overcome some day.

What did we learn from these dynamic leaders
Who fought for freedom the nonviolent way?
Did we learn wisdom? Did their wisdom teach us
So that we, too, can be leaders some day?

Let us now live the dream which they envisioned
And build a loving world of nonviolence;
Let's walk with God in these united nations
And let His love be our true defense.

We thank our great Creator for these legends
Who, through examples, showed the strength to love;
Let's live the dreamers dream of love's nonviolence
And build a glorious world of brotherly love.

Family caregiving experiences are geared to teach us that adversity is a spiritual gift. When we recognize the gift, as I like to say, it will help us to stop whining and start shining. Below is a song written by John and me to help us find inner peace.

STOP WHINING AND START SHINING!

Adversity is a hidden gift that deepens our insight
That God is always present in our world of day and night
When we in humble prayer express our gratitude to Him
His love within us lights our candles and we sing the hymn

—Refrain—
Out of darkness, God's light of love will shine
Shine into our kindness. What a joy divine!
Light your candles, you don't have to whine
Make your life a candlelight and you'll begin to shine.

Your caregiving world is Love's great blessing in disguise
When you put your trust in love, caregiving makes you wise!
With a heart of kindness, shine your candle through the night
You'll find joy and happiness in God's eternal light.

VISION FOUR
Take Your Candles, Light Up Your World

IN GRATITUDE TO OUR NURSES
Our nurses are God's candlelights, His angels of the earth, whose presence shines His light of love throughout the universe. —A. Johnson

NURSE VENITA HORSTMANN, OUR ACTIVITIES DIRECTOR

V for a **VESSEL**, she spreads loving care
E for her **EXCELLENCE** that's seen everywhere
N for her **NEWSLETTER**, uniquely done
I for her **IMAGE** her beauty has won
T for her **TEACHINGS** that make us feel smart
A for the **ANGEL** that dwells in her heart.

H for the **HAPPINESS** that shines in her smile
O for **OUTSTANDING, ...her** trademark profile
R for **REMARKABLE**...a gift she portrays
S for the **SWEETNESS** of her ardent ways
T for her **THOUGHTFULNESS** to those in her care
M for the **MAGIC** her guidance shares
A for the **ARTISTRY** her talent confers
N for her **NICENESS** in printing my verse
N for her **NICENESS** she's our favorite nurse.

We love **VENITA!** She's dear to our hearts!
Bravo, **VENITA!** The-state-of-the-arts!

NURSE MARYSE IS MS. SERIOUSNESS

Some patients call her Nurse Maryse
But I've a different name
Her seriousness stands out, you see
And this denotes her fame.
She's serious business in her walk
She's serious business in her talk
When she's on duty, no one balks
Her seriousness is no game.

She smiles a serious smile when things
Are moving as they should;
Co-workers know she pulls no strings,
Although they wish she would.
She's serious business in her work
She's serious business and she's perk
Perhaps there're those who want to smirk
But that would do no good.

For serious business is her style,
Her personality
She chats and laughs once in a while
She even laughs with me.
We all respect our nurse Maryse
Her seriousness is honesty
She uses her authority
With love and dignity.

When she's on duty you can bet
Good work is being done;
Her seriousness is stern but yet
Relaxes everyone.

The nurse aides love to do their best
And we, as patients, must confess
We love Nurse Maryse's seriousness
She's business, but she's fun.

'Twas the Creator who sent her
To serve this noble cause;
He made of her a serious nurse
To care for us because
She has the talent, and she's kind,
Even when she speaks her business mind;
Her business and beauty combined
Deserve our loud applause.

HERE COMES NURSE WILDA VALQUEZ, LPN

Wilda! She's like a breath of Spring
Kind, soft and gentle is her voice
I take the Calan that she brings
Without my usual fighting noise.

"Hi, Mr. Johnson," says her smile,
"It's time for your blood pressure pill."
I hesitate for just a while
And want to say "But I'm not ill."

Then, I recall the diagnosis
My MS stranger brought with him.
"Well okay, nurse, if you insist,"
I gently say without a whim.

"I want you to drink lots of fluid,"
Nurse Wilda says with cup in hand,
"'Cause, Mr. John, if you don't do it
You'll end up sick, you understand?"

She places Calan on my tongue
Then gives me fluid to wash it down
I feel contented, not high-strung
With that much water, one could drown.

Nurse Wilda smiles and says, "That's good!
You drank your fluid! I'm proud of you!"
I blush and whisper, "Perhaps I should
Be proud of MS Stranger, too."

Thank you, Nurse Wilda, you are grand
You show compassion to us all;
Nurses like you are in demand
You are an answer to God's call.

ABOUT NURSE BARBARA, OUR CNA

Barbara, ...our quiet CNA
Is Barbara-quiet in her Barbara-way,
She listens with both ears and eyes
To "No, No" voices and "Help me" cries.

When patient Olive Mahony pleaded
"Will you help me, nurse?" Barbara was needed
To help her walk her walker by
Ben's wheelchair in the hallway aisle.

Our Barbara, with her caring voice,
Smiled quietly into the tiny noise
And asked, "What is it, Olive dear?"
Says Olive, "Help me out of here!
Please, please, nurse will you help me please?"
Nurse Barbara's touch put her at ease.

"Oh, thank you nurse," Olive replied.
The caring touch exemplified
The kind of tender, loving care
That VA Nursing Homes do share.

But Olive's "Help me, please" persisted;
And Barbara quietly insisted
That she tell Barbara of her needs
And she would quietly help, indeed.

"Will you help me, nurse?" our Olive said.
Nurse Barbara smiled and shook her head
"It's your bedtime," Barbara declared,
"I can't let you go anywhere."

"But I'm not sleepy," Olive cried,
Her soft voice was a pleading sigh.
Though roommate Betty had gone to bed
Our Olive wanted to walk instead.

In quiet patients' loving care
Nurse Barbara, with her quiet air
Dressed Olive carefully for bed;
For quiet Barbara is quiet-bred.

When she's on duty you can bet
Her quietness earns our great respect.
Sometimes she helps put me to bed
After cold-like showers I sometimes dread.
She's very kind to all of us
That's why her kindness is "A-PLUS!"

Thank you, Nurse Barbara, for your gift
Of loving service on each shift
Thank you for kindnesses you give
Thank you for helping us to live
Thank you for tender nursing care
Thank you, Dear God, for Barbara dear.

"THANK YOU, NURSE CATHERINE"

She moves with gentleness and self-esteem
To do her many duties, some extreme
She does them all; and her work is supreme.
That's our Nurse Catherine!

She works with smiles throughout the busy day
Amid the cares that often underlay
Those "help me" cries we daily send her way.
"Thank you, Nurse Catherine!"

She'll pause to chat and laugh with us sometimes,
She makes us feel important at all times,
Especially during our daily eating times.
"Thank you, Nurse Catherine!"

She knows us by our first and our last names
But often uses titles just the same,
Sometimes she calls us those "sweetheart" nicknames.
"Thank you, Nurse Catherine."

At times she talks with patient Arianna Renn
Arianna's dimples ease into a grin,
They laugh a happy laugh and we join in.
"Thank you, Nurse Catherine"

Her laughter is like medicine, I confess,
But this she knows and always does her best
To bring us valued joy and happiness
"Thank you Nurse Catherine."
She is Rosanna and Lonie's dear mom
But at VA's Heartland she has become
A loving, caring nurse to everyone.
"Thank you, Nurse Catherine.

IN GRATITUDE TO NURSE NUBIA, CNA

Nubia! The tender voice of care,
She spreads love sunshine everywhere!
When she performs her daily tasks
She goes that extra mile unasked.
"Thank you, Nurse Nubia!"

She moves about the dining room
With lunch trays, napkins, folks and spoons
And helps the patients who're in need,
Some of them difficult to feed.
"Thank you, Nurse Nubia!"

She fed me 'till I finally learned.
I thanked her kindly in return.
With mushroom soup spilled in my lap
My chicken hit the floor "flip-flop!"

My roommate Ben said, "Nurse, come here,
Nurse Nubia rushed toward my chair
"Help roommate John, he dropped his meat,
Spilled mushroom soup all over his seat!"

When Nurse Nubia cleaned up my spills,
Our "Rose" shrieked. "Help! Help!" with a shrill.
Nurse Nubia rushed to help our Rose
Whose cottage cheese covered her nose.

"Why doesn't Rose eat with a spoon?"
Ben asked, and stared about the room.
Rose looked at Ben and said, "My Dear,
You keep your nose outta my affairs!"

"Now let's be nice," Nurse Nubia warned.
Rose answered, "Nice? Well I'll be darned!"
Nurse Nubia squeezed Rose's hand and smiled.
For "being kind" is Nubia's style.
We all thank you, Nurse Nubia.

At night and with a nursing aide
She tucks me safely into bed.
"Gracias," I say through sleepy eyes.
"Gracias!" she says and waves goodbye.

Thank you, Nurse Nubia, you are nice
Your nursing is like Paradise.

For works of kindness that you do
We thank VA and God for you!

NURSE WILMA CNA, OUR QUIET SMILE

Soft walking feet move swiftly by
I watch her quietly.
She smiles and goes about her duties
caring and bringing joy
to those for whom
she is responsible.
symbols of Love

Her kindness speaks
through deeds of deep concern.
And oftentimes I listen
wondering how does love
find expression.

She is my ardent nurse.
And from the depths of
higher understanding, she responds
with her heart to make my
life as comfortable
as her dedication.
With high respect, I
respond in kind;
but oftentimes my clouds of
yesterdays and
tomorrows sprinkle
rain. For this, I do
regret.

She understands. Yet I
dare not forget the
personality of Mysterious Stranger
who shares my space.
He fights and claws to
upstage my existence. But I dare not
retreat.

Thank you, Nurse Wilma, for your
gift of being...for you are
music sounds. Your caregiving has
shown me that love
finds its great expression
through kindness and concern.

TO OUR ARTHAL OF THE CUSTODIAL STAFF

Arthal Johnson is a smile that lights up every room
She is a precious angel...bedecked with mop and broom
She shines into the morning and throughout the livelong day
And we, in tribute, thank her in a very special way.

ABOUT OUR ARTHAL AND HER SPOTLESSNESS

Thank you, Mrs. Arthal and your staff
for keeping spick-and-span
The VA Nursing Home Floor 2 with your terrific plan
To make your work a masterpiece
With you and your staff's elbow grease
You are a conversation piece
A great custodian!

Your floors shine like a mirror;
Your furniture looks new;
And everything smells fresh and clean
in this Nursing Home -2.
In all your work your true love shines,
Your working staff is superfine!
We never hear you fuss and whine
In all that you pursue.

We all know that you love your work
And you do let us know
You "don't want anyone tramping over
Your wet, shiny clean floor.
You perch your hands upon your hips
Then pucker up your speechless lips
We run so fast we almost slip
When we hear your uproar!

We love the way you love your work.
It shines just like you do.
We love the neatness and clean smell
Of our Nursing Home-2
We love your caring attitude
Your friendliness, your fortitude,
Your kindness and your magnitude!
Mrs. Arthal, we thank you!

NURSE DEBORAH AND HER SPACE

Deborah's a very special nurse and she has special ways;
To know her is to love her for the frankness she displays.
She speaks out with authority

And lets her inner mind convey
The thoughts that always seem to say
"I'm master of my space!"

She works with great authority in Nursing Home Floor-2;
She cares about her patients and does what she has to do.
"Patients are my priority,
And my responsibility,"
She frankly said with honesty
But this, we always knew.

She speaks out for her patients, and keeps them nice and clean;
She showers them and combs their hair in her daily routine.
Her voice, sometimes forceful and strong,
Demands that they help her along
To help her help them all day long
She works like a machine.

Her daughter is a college grad, I said, "Deborah, Bravo!
If she's as smart and kind as you,
you've earned the highest score!
And now I understand your ways
And how you can control your space
You're filled with God's amazing grace
Deborah, you're great to know.

Housekeeping staff has labeled you "a serious business" girl;
To love you is to know you in your Deborah Williams world.
Sometimes you make us very glad
And some of us a little mad
But we all love you dear comrade,
You are a precious pearl!

You are a pearl to all of us if only we would see
The lessons we all gain from your firm personality.
You make us practice what we preach
Unknowingly, that's what you teach
You help us learn through your outreach
To thank humanity.

VISION FIVE
Candlelights from the Resident Patients' and Caregivers' Worlds

By Patient John Johnson
and wife/caregiver/ghostwriter Alice

No one has ever seen God; but when we love one another,
God lives in us, and His love is made complete in us.
—1 John 4:12

Prelude

Astounded by the many deeds of kindness and the brightness of the candlelights that surrounded them, and the many resident patients and their candlelights, the awakened traveler made the sign of the cross and knelt in silent prayer:

Kind Master, I thank you for the joy of talking with my husband, John, and various patients who voice their sentiments with your prophet St. Paul who said: "I have learned, in whatsoever state I am in, therewith to be content."

Thank you from the depths of my heart for revealing to me that our ailing brothers and sisters are here to teach us the wisdom of love, compassion and service. I am grateful for the ability to put John's and my thoughts in poetic verse, and for the opportunity to be his hands and share his insights, thoughts and feelings from a broader prospective.

I am especially grateful for the joy each poem bought to the patients, their families and friends as they listened with childlike smiles and appreciation, knowing that they all are loved, appreciated and respected. John and I saw the child within each patient, and that child is an expression of your love.

With these many experiences of love in action, we will

always feel as one in the heart of all creation. May we always keep these symbols of love and these attitudes of gratitude in our spiritual awareness. Amen.

About our "ROSE"

(Our nursing home patient
and former public school English teacher)

Rose, Rose, our precious Rose
Her "Help, Help, Help" through music flows.

And with her tiny feet she goes
Courageously through Heartland's doors.
O'er purple carpets, polished floors
Her wheelchair quietly takes our Rose.

In the soft magic of her eyes
Her "help, help, help" conveys her cries;
A kind nurse aide quickly replies,
"My dearest Rose, please tell me why
Do you cry 'Help' when we pass by?"

To this, Rose quickly clarifies
Her "help, help, help" to passers-by;
"You nurses seem preoccupied
With other patients and their cries.
So this is why I understand
You can't always give me a hand."

We smiled, agreeing with our Rose;
She smiled and gave us an encore
Of "Help, Help, Help." We all adore
Our precious Rose, we love her so.

OUR VETERAN ,"BEN," ENVISIONED

Envisioned Ben,
My nursing home friend,
We chat of places we have been.
He was a National Guard major
Stationed in New York, he did say.

He talked of army regiments
And places some of us were sent
To serve our country honorably
And help defend our USA.

Ben has a most exciting life
With lovely Molly as his wife.
The two of them took many trips
On many planes and many ships.

Ben and his Molly worked hand-in-hand;
Life's joyful blessings at their command.
They had a Denver pharmacist friend
Whom they both visited now and then.

This wealthy friend had a drug store
Where Ben and Molly would often go.

Ben said, "My Molly and I would dwell
At Denver's Cow Place Hotel."
Sometimes they went to Colorado Springs
To see the many lovely things
The Indians made and tourists bought
In Pike's Peak where they often stopped.

When World War II came to an end
They kept in touch with their dear friend.
Ben and his loving wife moved East
Their marriage was a lover's feast.

They traveled North, South, East and West
Then one day she laid down to rest.
Ben speaks of her with so much love
She'll always be his dear beloved.

Said he, "My Molly still lights up my world;
We met when she was just a girl."
I share with Ben my army days,
That brought me to this VA space.

I was a sergeant in Korea
I sorta liked that new career.

Then multiple sclerosis came aboard
And brought along its MS sword.

It chopped away my healthy life
But Love had given me a wife.
Who gave me spiritual support,
Now caregiving's her favorite sport.

Whenever my Alice visits me
We both go on a writing spree;
We talk with Ben remembering
Our days in Colorado Springs.

My wife has lots of family there
On visits she pulls up a chair.

Ben shares the happenings of his world,
Experiences of his life unfurl.

"My Denver friend has a 'spirits' store,"
Ben said to us, then added more.
"But in those days when times were rough
Drug stores were licensed to sell that stuff.
My Denver friend was very smart
He sold the stuff right from the start
"Made lots of money; the guy got rich!"
"Got rich?" I said and scratched my itch.

"Sure, he got rich," Ben laughed and said.
I scratched again my itching head.

I said, "Sounds like my money plan,
'To make what-you-can as fast-as-you-can
Then can-the-can ,and sit-on-your-can.'"
Ben chuckled, "That sounds just like my man."

"But, Ben, did he slow down?" I asked.
Ben shook his head. I knew the rest.
"But we had fun," Ben said and grinned,
"Yes, Molly and me and our Denver friends."

"Write that down, Alice," I told my wife.
"I'll write a poem about Ben's life."
My Alice said, "Let's ask the nurse,
But, John, you'd better ask Ben first."

To this Ben said in quick reply,
"Why ask my nurse, John, Alice? Why?"

I shrugged, then spooned into my beans,
"Because we'd hate to come between
The nursing profile you have here
in VA's great circle of care."

Ben said, "The idea sounds like fun;
I'll read it carefully when you're done."

My Alice's first draft had mistakes.
Ben read and said, "For goodness sakes,
You have me mixed up with Cliff, but then
Perhaps you'll write my poem again."

Ben made corrections and she wrote.
I laughed, "She can't read her own notes.
"Her scribbling's mixed with Gregg's Shorthand."
Ben said, "Ah-h-h, now I understand
Why Alice didn't get it right
Her scribbling, John, is outta sight!"

"Back off, you guys," my Alice said;
She jiggled my ear and squeezed my head.

Ben laughed then spoke of Denver times,
And I programmed them in my mind.

The three of us did chat away
With Ben we travel vicariously.

We're thankful for good vets like Ben
He's such a pleasant, loving friend.
Our VA nursing home to me
Is quite a pleasant place to be.

Thanks for this nursing home, VA
Thanks for the kindness you portray.
Our attitude of gratitude
Has now become our spiritual food.

CHATTING WITH WAR VETERAN "CLIFF"

I eat with Cliff at table three
I chat with him, he chats with me
Through happy voices at mealtime.
He speaks as clearly as he can
Of his Michelle and Corrie Anne
With Cliff, it's sharing-time.

He speaks of his devoted wife
She is the essence of his life
Who loves her Cliff sincerely.
He said Eurika is her name
And all through life she is the same
That's why he loves her dearly.

The other day Cliff said to me
He once did household carpentry
For a construction firm.
He laid both wooden and tile floors
All kinds of work for the indoors
'Till nature took its turn.

Yes, nature brought him to VA
Where angels care for him each day
With tender, loving care;
Through kind caregivers he receives

The kind of service that relieves
The burdens he once feared.

'Tis fun to talk with Cliff each day
We share our happy thoughts this way
Over breakfast, lunch and dinner.
With his Michelle and Corrie Anne
And wife Eurika, he's quite a man
Our Cliff's a happy winner.

About Our "JAMES FERRALL"
(The VA and Heartland Nursing Home)

Often I eat with James at dinnertime
We talk of good ol' working days sometimes.
"What was your job before you came in here?"
I asked James as he stirred in his wheelchair.

"Was a 'Lieutenant Detective' on the Beach.
I worked there thirty years," he said and reached
for his tall glass of cold cranberry juice,
and spoke of his kind loving wife, Lucia.

"She bought me here because I had a stroke,"
he said, and then continued unprovoked.
"Yes, three days after Hurricane Andrew
I had a stroke! 'twas nothing I could do.
We'd moved to a motel 'cause the hurricane
Had blown our house away in Key Biscayne."

"And your Miami Beach detective job
Was taken by Andrew who liked to rob,"

I said, "'cause Andrew robbed me of my home.
But you lost job, house and your honey-comb.
'Tis nice your Lucia keeps you at VA
Where you'll recuperate first-hand, I'd say."

"Your Lucy said you both have lovely kids."
James smiled and said, "We've three, and heaven forbid.
They've all grown up now and I'm glad to say
They're doing fine." He nodded happily.

"I bet one is a lawyer," our Ben said,
To this James stared at him, nodding his head.
"That's great!" I said to my cranberry juice,
"Tell him to sue Mom Nature for child abuse.
Her Andrew took James' health, good job and house.
We veterans need to be like Mighty Mouse."
James pantomimed his hands 'round Andrew's neck.
"He'll bite us both," I said, "Andrew's a snake.

"He took us from our wives, James, they're alone;
He took your health, your job, totaled our home!
But let's thank God that Andrew brought us here."
James smiled into sweet music in the air.

God speaks through our experiences to us
To say "Thank you" to others is a must.
We must be grateful for each kindly deed
For we are vessels helping those in need.

Tho' we're disabled we can still be kind
by saying 'Thank You' we are bound to find
That being grateful gives us joy inside
So, let's be grateful, happy, satisfied.

Both Ben and James with nodding heads agreed
That being grateful is a must, indeed.

About "OUR JENNIE GRESSETT"
(At Heartland of Kendall Nursing Home)

Our Jennie, with "sweet Jennie-talk"
And matching outfits, likes to walk
In slow pace up/down Heartland's halls
Of inlaid carpets, hand-railed walls.

Her friendly chatter, dimpled smile
Portray love feelings, Jennie-style;
With nurse aides Joyce and Manie's skills
"Jen" eats and talks without food spills.

"Finish your food, Jen," the nurse aides said.
But Jenny, dressed in fancy red,
Softly replied, "I'll do my best."
She did, and gave her voice a rest.

Nurse Aide Myrlande came to assist,
Cut Jenny's meat like a chef-artist.
"Eat your food, Jen," she said and left.
"Thank you!" said Jen, as she fed herself.

"When I went shopping," Jennie teased,
"I bought all these, and these, and these!"
My Alice asked, 'Where, at the store?"
Envisioning Lucinne's "No, no, no!"

Through Jennie's tender talk talk talk
Kind nurse aides waited without a squawk;
Jen's friendly chatter lit the room
'Till Mario came with sweeping broom.

"I guess it's clean-up time," Jen said.
Our Mario smiled, nodding his head.
Our Jennie finished her food and then
Her sweet, soft chatter began again.

She looked around, her friends had left
Louise, Olive, Anna, and Bess,
Pauline, Etta, Hazel, and Ben
Ariane, Helen, Stella. But when?

Even Julia, Irene, Margaret, and Cliff,
Mary, Evelyn, and the other Cliff,
Gertrude, Franklin, Edith and those.
When did they ease through dining room doors?

"I'd better leave now," our Jennie said,
"Good Lord, it'll soon be time for bed!"
Jennie left, changed outfits, and did her deed,
Pushing wheelchair friends that seemed in need.

"Be careful, Jennie," Nurse Maryse warned;
Then moved Margaret as Jen looked on.
"I want to help you all," Jen cried.
"I understand," Nurse Maryse replied.

"Our staff is here for everyone,"
Nurse Maryse said in serious tongue.

"So let them do their job, sweetheart."
For serious business is Maryse's art.

Jen saw a wheelchair friend at rest
And felt her friend was in distress.
"I'll push you to your room," she said.
"The nurses will put you to bed."

"Look, Jen, you've both socks on one foot,"
Our Nurse Aide Barbara said, "So put
One sock on your left foot, Jen, dear.
No barefootedness, sweetheart, in here!"

"I know," our Jennie said and paused,
"I put both on one foot because
It is my business and not yours!"
Nurse Barbara smiled at Jennie's toes.

"We're here to help you, my dear Jen,"
Nurse Barbara said, kneading her chin.
Jennie replied, "I understand...
And Thank You!" She squeezed Barbara's hand.

Jen, thus, continued to push her friend
And help her move toward the end
Of the long hallway to her room
Then smiled a smile brightly illumined.

"Jen's always helping in some way,"
Nurse Barbara said, moving Jen's food tray.
Jen's acts of kindness are so sweet
We call her precious and unique.

Nurse Wilda said, "Jen's a delight!
Sometimes she walks the hall at night."
The nurses show true love for Jen
For Heartland's staff is our true friend.

Symbols of love our Jennie gives
Thanksliving is the life she lives;
She loves all people we are told,
For love paints beauty in her soul.

We're grateful for Jennie Gressett
She is a candlelight at best;
She creates her own happiness
Our Jennie in the bright red dress.

ABOUT OUR "MARGARET"

(80-year old patient and former department store division manager)

'Twas Margaret who helped write Natasha's poem
She gave us rhyming words and we moved on
Today we're at a party and there's noise
In spite of it we hear each other's voice.

"What can we rhyme with Heartland?" I did ask.
And Margaret stared at me, her thoughts unmasked;
With outstretched hands she whispered, "Understand."
Yes, that's the word that rhymes with our Heartland."

I smiled and nodded to my wife and said,
"Write that down, Alice." She wrote it and read.

We listened to each word and Margaret asked,
"Do you think writing poetry is a task?"

"Not really," Alice said, and I agreed.
So Margaret helped according to our need.
"What rhymes with the word 'sound?'" we asked and stared.
When Margaret said "around," my Alice cheered.

Then Margaret added sentences that rhymed.
My Alice wrote them down in scheduled time.
My Alice said, "Gee, Margaret, you're a poet!"
"Oh, no," said Margaret, "That's the poem you wrote."

"But you helped; us!" I said and sipped my juice,
Yet trying to convince her was no use.
She didn't want the credit and insisted
We give ourselves the credit. We resisted.

"We'll write a poem about the help you gave,"
I said into loud music and her wave.
"Oh no," she said, then added a half smile,
"This kind of party is a little wild."

We broke in laughter, Margaret, Al and I.
"But this is fun," Al said, "Do you see why?"
"They're having fun," said Margaret with a smile.
"This kind of music just isn't my style."

But Margaret is creative, this we know.
Perhaps one day and at another show
We'll chat with her and write down what she said,
Put it to poetry and then have it read.
It's fun to chat with others and make friends

We're thankful for friendships that never end
Let's make spreading our love a major trend..

AN ODE TO MY FORMER NURSING HOME ROOMMATE, "ALBERT"

(Albert was a pilot in the Korean War)

Where did he go, this spirit of divineness?
His name was Albert, my roommate and friend.
We think of him, endowed with human kindness,
His energy, oh where did it ascend?

He left one morning in the month of July;
Paramedics came to take Albert away.
We paused and stared, then waved a prayerful goodbye
And prayed that he'd come back to us one day.

Our minds recalled his kind and gentle manner
He thanked the nurses, even in his pain.
He'd call the nurses, and they'd quickly answer.
Though he was ill, he seldom would complain.

He once gave me his soft food in my hunger
Because my aching jaw was wracked with pain.
I'll never forget his kindness, and I wonder
Was he God's angel on this earthly plane?

I'm sure he was and I'm so glad I met him
He spoke with love of friends and family,
From planet earth the angels came to get him
And take him home into eternity.

His life was filled with meaning and with purpose
And flowed in beauty, wisdom, love and grace.
We know his spirit is forever with us
Because his soul has found its resting place.

We are but energy, his life has taught us,
And energy can never be destroyed.
We'll always "be," 'twas nature who begot us;
We are eternal; we live in the Lord.

Yes, we are one in spirit and in purpose
To love and help each other and to share;
So, like our Albert, let us thank our nurses,
and thank VA for this circle of care.

About Our "SYLVIA BERSON"

(HRC resident and former public school teacher)

She's friendly and she loves to smile
She talks with anyone.
She plays Bingo with friends downstairs,
She lives with friends who live upstairs,
She loves them all, they're hers and theirs,
'Cause Sylvia loves fun.

She dances like a dancing pro
When Don and Amy play.
She sings along with Sammy, too;
She swings, and waltzes with the crew.
According to our interview
She's always been that way.

"My husband, Ralph, wrote music,"
Our Sylvia said and smiled.
"I have one son and several grands,
A lovely daughter-in-law, Susan.
They visit me here at Heartland.
Each one's my precious child."

If you know Sylvia, you'll admit
That she is loving, too!
She's proud of her kind family,
And speaks of it so interestingly;
We'll write her story joyfully
one day to share with you.

About "HAROLD", MY NEW ROOMMATE

(A professional actor and a Korean War veteran patient at Heartland Nursing Home)

Part 1

When roommate Albert quietly went to his eternal home,
Administration, caring
knew that I was all alone.

They moved me into Harold's room where I'd have company;
I thanked them for this kind gesture
and knew I'd love my stay.

It seemed that all my past roommates had eminent domain.
And even Harold, my good friend,
who welcomed me right in.

The nurses kindly moved my clothes and me in Harold's room.
My Alice came to see me but
our joy soon turned to gloom.

When we saw paramedics taking Harold from his bed,
we asked, "What's wrong with Harold?"
and the nurses kindly said,
"Our Harold fell and hurt his hip,
and now he is in pain.
He must go to the hospital,
but he'll be back again."

"The hospital," my Alice shrieked,
then looked at me wide-eyed.
I knew what she was thinking, so I suddenly replied,
"Our Harold will be back real soon,
you must believe this truth.
My other roommates that went home
did not have Harold's youth."
She stared at me in total shock; surprised that I recalled
that five roommates boarded their planes
'cause death's bright angel called.

Nurse Maryse said, "They're taking Harold just to get x-rays.
He should be back here at Heartland
in just a couple days."

Al scratched into her curly perm,
then looked at me and smiled.
"Oh yes, our Harold's coming back
in just a little while."

Part 2

A few days later, Harold came; and, oh boy, was I glad!
He is the first verbal roommate
that I have ever had.
He talked of sports, current events,
we were surprised to learn
that we're both from Ohio
with memories to confirm.

We're Catholics, and artists,
and we're both Columbus Knights.
Harold performed in stage plays
Like the ones Al and I write.

Part 3

'Twas "The House Without Children" in which he played
a poor butler's son, but wise
Who worked for a rich couple with one child
all beautiful and sad-eyed.

The butler, so blessed with his wall-to-wall-kids,
was as poor as he could be.
But the love that he shared in his dirt-poor home
made them spiritually rich and wealthy.

"I'll bring you some pictures of that great play,"
said Harold from his wheelchair.
"Gee, Harold, I'd love to see them," I replied,
brushing Grecian Formula hair.

When we spoke of the Knights of Columbus, he said,
"John, I am a Fourth Degree Knight!"
"Well congratulations!" I said to him.
"Harold, that is the highest height!"

He smiled and nodded a "Thank You" to me
as we both continued to talk.
"I'm a Third-Degree Knight," I said to him,
"'Cause MS wouldn't let me walk."

We watched the Cleveland Indians' game
when his Margaret stopped by that day.
We three talked of the performing arts
and spoke of Don and Amy.

"That Don and Amy are great," Harold said,
"They certainly can perform!"
To this, both Margaret and I agreed
and applauded this nursing home.

"Those songs bring back sweet memories,"
Harold said without a doubt.
"My wife and I would sing them all
Whenever we'd go out."
"Especially songs like All of Me,
Daisy and Mary Anne.
They're typical of the fun we had
at home before VA's Heartland.

Part 4

But I am so glad that Administration
is blessed with the keen insight

to keep our musical souls alive
with memories that enlight.

We're glad that the enlightened heart and mind
are nourished at VA's Heartland.
And we are grateful for the staff
that fashioned this command.

I'm thankful for my roommate, Harold;
for he is a world of fun.
I thank Heartland for the insight,
of my social need for someone.

"Being all alone is unhealthy,"
Nurse Maryse had said to me.
So they put me and my illness in Harold's room
'cause it's medical therapy.

THREE CHEERS FOR CLIFFORD YOUNG

A vessel of love is Cliff Young,
My good ol' army friend.
We sometimes talk of army days
In army talk and army ways
When thoughts of army life ablaze
Such memories never end.
They're memories that love transcends

Our Clifford once lived in Brownsville
Of Miami, Northwest
He worked for Joe Caleb, his friend, a young man

A Black union leader who took a great stand
That put more money in poor men's hands
Whose courage stood the test.
He was the union's best!

A center was built in Joe's honor
When he was shot to death
Yes, Caleb Community Center is huge
Cost millions of dollars 'cause he was no stooge
His multiethnic union was not like ol' scrooge
We don't know who took Joe's breath.
Can love for one's neighbors cost death?

Cliff speaks with interest of his life
That comes back like a song
Like Joe, he's a kind and gentle man
A symbol of love who lends a hand
To many vets here at VA's Heartland.
We thank you, Clifford , you're strong.
Keep loving and you can't go wrong.

OUR SCHOLARLY VETERAN FRANKLIN JOHNSON

(A former executive director of a huge business firm)

He wears his dignity with style;
and greets you with a quiet smile
He's quiet and sometimes versatile
He's scholarly Franklin Johnson.

He reads good books and magazines
and chats with others in between.
Watches PBS on

TV screen
That's our Franklin Johnson.

He shares news articles with me,
MS research, especially,
"And Betaseron's research,"
he said," has been approved."
He takes his MS like a champ.
His courage is a lighted lamp
that often helps us to revamp
our positive attitude.

He sometimes likes to eat alone.
He talks with friends by telephone.
Here at Heartland he feels
at home.
We love our Franklin Johnson.

OUR DEAR FRIEND "ANGELES WAY"

(A resident and former college professor of English)

(1)
Our Angeles Way loves to get
mail
as most people like to do.
Now she's at Heartland with good friends
who love to get mail, too.

(2)
Especially Harold, a gentle
man
who eats with her each day.

And Margaret, too, a beautiful friend
who's kind in every way.

(3)
Our Angeles is quite lovely,
too.
We love her very much.
And we, the sweethearts of Heartland,
do honor her as such.

So, here's a poem, a special
poem
in Angeles' mail today
that speaks of love; of Heartland's love,
of our precious Angeles Way.

VISION SIX

Candlelights from VA'S Recreational Therapy World

There are two ways to live your life. One is as though nothing is a miracle. The other is as though everything is a miracle. —Albert Einstein

THE DON AND AMY SHOW

(Fun at VA Vets Heartland of Kendall Nursing Home to enhance interpersonal and social skills)

Did you see 'the Don and Amy Show'
at the Nursing Home yesterday?
We had a good time "singing along!"
That's all I need to say.

Nine residents had birthdays,
I'll try to name a few:
Our Sylvia Berson, Irving Cowan,
Rose Angel and Savitz, too.

Our Helen Warner, Helen Proctor,
James Humphrey, also,
including our Jean Herskwitz,
who actually stole the show.

We all sang "Happy Birthday"
to this nine-member team,
born in the ninth month of the year,
September's Kings and Queens.

We danced to Amy's "Stardust."
My roommate, Harold, sang.

Our Margaret, Ben and Angeles Way
applauded everything!

When Amy danced with Kilborn and me
in our wheelchairs, 'twas fun.
Her "Let me Call you Sweetheart"
made us want to say "WELCOME!"

Her "Maryanne," "All of Me," and
"Whatever Will Be, Will Be,"
Her "Molly and Me," "Daisy, Daisy,"
made us feel fancy free.

Our Amy, in glittering attire,
danced with us all, I'd say
We really enjoyed our singing along
with talented Don and Amy!

We're grateful for our nursing home
that makes our spirits glow
Our attitude is gratitude
for the Don and Amy show.

Thank you, VA! Thank you Heartland!
for teaching social skills
We're made to enjoy other wonderful folks
It's therapy for our ills.

When we respect, appreciate,
and love our neighbors all,
regardless of their faith or race,
we'll love this spiritual call.

Let's learn from Don and Amy's show
How we can sing along
And our multicultural world
can be one peaceful song.

ALIVE WITH SAMMY'S MUSIC

We had a party here today...on August twenty four.
'Twas Hurricane Andrew's first birthday;
just thought you oughta know.

It was a way of celebrating that we are alive
in spite of Andrew's destruction, our Heartland has survived.

Yes, it was just one year ago in nineteen ninety-two
when Heartland's staff protected us from, Hurricane Andrew.

That vicious storm destroyed South Dade
and wrecked Kendall's Heartland.
But Heartland's Board reached out in love,
rebuilt this wonderland.

Therefore today we celebrate in gratitude because
our love expressed in music is an endless applaud.

Venita, our activity director and her skillful staff,
Natasha and Gisela, planned this fun on our behalf.

Their leadership's dynamic, and they bring us lots of fun.
Their "Sing Along With Sammy" is enjoyed by everyone.

We clap our hands and pat our feet to music Sam provides.
We sing along with Sammy as we sway from side to side.

When Sammy played "Blue Heaven,"
Sylvia clapped and sang along,
with Margaret, Mary, Clara, Gertrude, Sadie going strong.

The nurses: Agnes, Carolyn, Gail, Raymona and the rest
applauded with the patients,
and brought smiles to the depressed.

As private nurse Raymona danced with Ben and moved about,
then Nurse Julia brought patient Jean her medicine en route.

Camille Crooke fed Jean Sorcher a sandwich as she danced,
while Sammy sang "Match Maker,"
pulling up his sagging pants.

We knew that our leadership, in skillful formula,
had planned this "Sing Along" for us and folks like Angela,
Our Angela was hooked up to her feeding tube, you see,
but Sammy's music awakened her to pleasant memories.

His "Happy Days Are Here Again"
was sung with so much joy,
our world of memories came alive,
and we all screamed, "Oh Boy!"

With Sammy's rich and powerful voice,
our feelings came alive,
and songs like our "Sweet Georgia Brown"
was such a power drive!

When Gail St. Phillip, LPN, joined in the clapping fun,
our counselor Madeline danced about, smiling with everyone.

Said Carolyn Anthony, CNA, "Look at Clara McPhee!
She's always sound asleep but now she's wide awake!
Oh Gee!"
When Sammy's "On The Road Again" sent us into the shakes,
the rhythm brought us to our feet, we all felt wide awake!

Then Pauline Weiss and Etta showed polished long fingernails,
and sung their "Side By Side" with Sammy;
they could not be still

"Over the Rainbow" Sam took us into his "Freedom Land,"
Where we looked "Over a Four-Leaf Clover"
right here in wonderland.

And now we're "Sitting-On-top-Of-The-World"
and moving right along
just singing, dancing, clapping, prancing to each happy song.

When Nurses Wilda and Maryse walked in,
they paused awhile
"Good Heaven's!" said Nurse Mryse
in her cute and serious smile,
"What's going on in here?" she asked into the happy noise.
But music from the joyful singing drowned out her voice.

Nurse Wilda said, "Mrs. Johnson, I saw YOU on TV...YOU!"
The national news on TV told of Alice and Andrew.

But Andrew's lessons and VA blessings
brought me to Heartland;

and to this great "Circle of Love"
to SING ALONG WITH SAM!

We all thank Heartland for this fun and for activities
that keep our spiritual world alive with fun things such as this!

We thank our nursing staff for joining us in dance and song,
and thank Administration
who, through Andrew, stood so strong.

Our attitude is gratitude, a lesson Oprah taught.
'Twas she who made us look inside
our feelings and our thoughts.

Showers of blessings surfaced in our journal writing world
Feelings that come from being grateful is a precious pearl.

Love always finds expression
through our kindness and concern.
Thus, "singing along with Sammy"
helps us patients love and learn.
To say " thank you" to nursing homes like VA and Heartland
Where their kindness and love reflect that God is in command.

In Summary for the Poetic Family Caregiver

ART AND THE HUMAN SPIRIT

By Alice W. Johnson

The love of God is the highest good we humans can attain!
Let art bespeak this good in all its forms to yet explain
The thoughts and feelings of the human spirit at its best
Through love's artistic geniuses whose minds endure the test.

An artist feels the depth of love that flows from humankind
And uses art to share deep feelings of the human mind.
He paints the human spirit at its best and at its worse;
For life's experiences can be a blessing and a curse.

Art forms bespeak the good in men like Gandhi and like King
Revealing their true love of God...the highest good attained.
Art forms bespeak the feelings of suffering humanity
Through art we see love's highest good
that godliness portrays.

Art teaches us that love's the greatest creation of life
And that the human spirit can endure both calm and strife.
Art forms reveal that we all have a blessing and a cross
Divine love is our blessing, without it, we suffer loss.

Art teaches us that life's, indeed, a mystery to be lived
Let us like Jesus, Gandhi, King embrace life as we give
Our varying talents to the cause of universal peace,
With social justice, brotherly love we'll paint a masterpiece!

Life's a series of multi-problem-solving situations;
Let's paint our multi-cultural world
with love through race relations.
And let our human spirits, thus, artistically unfold
That through our art we learn
that love paints beauty in the soul.

About "Chicken Soup for the Veteran's Soul" and Family Caregiving

Enlightened by the many artistic stories in Canfield, Hansen and Slagter's *Chicken Soup for the Veteran's Soul,*

John and I purchased several copies of the book from Barnes and Noble bookstore and gave them to the nursing home veterans as treasured gifts. The veterans were astounded. They love the interesting stories. In the future, John and I will write their captivating responses in poetic verse.

Unfortunately, the VA Medical Center's Canteen does not carry the books. The store manager said that selling books is no longer their policy. How strange and unfair to the disabled veterans who are VA nursing home residents and who have served our country with courage. Inasmuch as we are approaching another shocking conflict and are relying upon our courageous armed forces who are the caregivers for our country, we need to make the books available to our VA nursing home residents "to stir the pride and honor the courage of our veterans" and us family caregivers who are still happily married to them.

In the past, the VA Canteen has sold John's books and my books. How could the manager deny the veterans the joy of reading a book about veterans, written by veterans for veterans and their families?

The veterans at the VA Medical Center found it interesting to know that the *Chicken Soup for the Veteran's Soul* contains the true-life experiences of extraordinary men and women in every branch of service. They learned that each of the people in the book were instrumental in changing the course of history through their acts of valor in World War II, Korea, the Vietnam War and the Persian Gulf War.

Like our veterans, we family caregivers can begin being instrumental in changing the course of history through deeds of kindness in a world now torn with horrible and heartbreaking experiences of man's inhumanity to man, and the frightening threat of major wars. We can share wisdom gained from family caregiving to help transform the world by writing our experiences that will help others spiritually...

1. Develop a kind attitude
2. Learn to speak kindly
3. Perform deeds of kindness

Today's World Needs Kindness

Today, especially, the world needs kindness. By being kind, we have the power to make the world a happier place in which to live.

The world is unkind only for the lack of kindness in the individuals who live in it. It is, therefore, very important that we as family caregivers share the real meaning of this kindness and continue to practice what we already know from experience.

There is no greater awakening to kindness than that which has its inspiration through the experiences of family caregiving. Our disabled loved ones, many of whom have served in the armed forces, have taught us this wisdom. In addition, our loved ones have taught that there is no more genuine kindness than that which has its inspiration through the grace of God in the perfect fulfillment of His greatest law, the law of love: "Love the Lord your God with all your heart, soul, strength and mind, and your neighbor as yourself."

When we are kind, we put others in the place of ourselves. Self-love becomes unselfishness.

Kindness is God in the act of creation and the constant preservation of the world in existence. From divine kindness flows the powers and the blessings of all created kindness. With this created kindness, we family caregivers and our loved ones can write volumes of poems expressing our gratitude to those nursing staff members and resident patients who touch lives and lift spirits.

Let us continue to write in our gratitude journals, using prose and poetry to find the light within and light up our world of family caregiving. Using our spiritual keys of (1) writing for Him, (2) gratitude, (3) kindness, (4) touching lives, lifting spirits, and (5) poetry therapy, we can avoid caregiver-burnout, promote inner peace and, using Spiritual Key #6, share this wisdom with the world to help transform it through kindness. Let us, in the words of Ernest Shurtleff, courageously say: "Through days of preparation, Thy grace has made us strong; and now, O King Eternal, we lift our battle song" as we shine our candles of kindness into the spiritual world.

Spiritual Key # 6

Candlelights for the Spiritual World

The spirit of man is the candle of the Lord.
— Proverbs 20:27.
It is better to light a candle than to curse the darkness.
—A Chinese proverb.

THE SPIRITUAL JOURNEY WITH CANDLELIGHTS

Live as children born in the light. Light produces all kindness, goodness, justice and truth. —Ephesians 5:8-9

Prelude

In the quietness of the soul, the awakened traveler lit a candle. Then staring pensively into its flame, she began to meditate, feeling humbled and thankful that the inquiring voice throughout the discussion was representative of all family caregivers throughout the world.

"Kind Master," she said silently, "we thank You for awakening us through caregiver/patient responsibilities to see, experience, feel and appreciate the spirit of lovingkindness in all your creation. How can I now summarize for others the many lessons of kindness my disabled brother has taught me?"

"My child," the kind Master whispered, "in the quietness of your mind, let the universe speak to you, for wisdom is its crown. You must silently listen, then light your candle and join your disabled brother in your missions to creatively spread the message of kindness throughout the world."

Candlelights of Kindness: The Gifts of Family Caregiving

Once upon a murderous windstorm called Hurricane Andrew, my husband said into my panic fears, "God is in everything and everything is in God. Why are you so afraid?" I was overwhelmed by the thought, but embittered by the question. I knew it would take tremendous growth for me to accept his powerful statement about God. I often wondered why did God give him so much wisdom and gave me the heavy cross of long-term family caregiving.

Well, I soon learned to listen to my husband because according to the silent voice within me, I was told that my husband and his good buddy, multiple sclerosis, came to teach me how to live God's treasury of virtues. When I discovered that these virtues would protect me from the "murderous windstorms" of life and of caregiver-burnout, and would bless me with the gifts of spiritual growth and inner peace, I whispered, "Shun not the struggle, face it; 'tis God's gift. Be strong!"

Family caregiving experiences, gratitude journal writing, the VA Medical Center and Nursing Home, and a host of professionals and paraprofessionals provided that spiritual growth through deeds of kindness. They were candlelights! Through them, I was able to see that *God is in everything and everything is in God.*

On the spiritual journey, my husband and I learned that a miracle is a universal blessing from our kind Master, and that miracles should inspire gratitude, not awe. On the family caregiving journey, we learned that everything that comes from love is a miracle, and miracles occur naturally as expressions of lovingkindness.

The statement, "God is in everything I see," awakened us to look at all things with love, kindness, appreciation and open-mindedness. We learned from our many spiritual leaders that love cannot be far behind a heart that is kind and thankful, and a mind that is grateful. Life taught us that our kind Master enters easily into our hearts when we love and are kind and grateful, for these are the prerequisites for our returning home to Him.

Our spiritual keys of family caregiving, if followed, will help avoid caregiver- burnout and promote inner peace. By writing meditatively from our world of family caregiving, we are awaken to the spiritual messages taught by our disabled loved ones. We *feel* the love within us that lights our candles of gratitude and kindness, enabling us to grow spiritually as we touch lives and lift spirits.

May we all, as candlelights, project the spirit of kindness that will forever be a pathway to God's love, wisdom and abundant life. In this twenty-first century, we family caregivers can enlarge our territories by using our candles to light up the world around us, promoting social justice, universal peace and brotherly love...one kind deed at a time.

Epilogue

As a more awakened traveler, accustomed to the tradition of writing through the pain and suffering that stem from family caregiving experiences and finding the spiritual message that enhances inner peace, I have been writing and rewriting this book through the tremendous grief and pain of coping with the terrorists attacks that sent us into shock. Oftentimes, tears blinded my vision and I could barely see the computer keyboard or read what I was writing. But I continued writing through the pain because it was the best way I could meditate prayerfully and control my thoughts, feelings and actions. The following quotation written by Graham Green seems an idealistic explanation for my reactions.

> *Writing is a form of therapy; sometimes I wonder how all those who do not write, compose or paint can manage to escape the madness, the melancholia, the panic fear which is inherent in the human situation.*

Using my therapy to escape the feelings of shock, dismay and anger of what had happened on September 11, 2001, I went on a writing spree and compiled these spiritual keys to share what many long-term family caregivers, I am sure, have also experienced.

We know from our human experiences of family

caregiving that *kindness* is, indeed, the true universal religion. Kindness is spiritual.

Knowing that in the midst of adversities we family caregivers are always arriving at higher levels of spiritual growth, we can use our spiritual keys to continue life's journey of spreading love through deeds of kindness.

Our wonderful President George W. Bush wants us to continue using our various talents to lift humanity. Adhering to his wise counseling that dried my tears, I envisioned authoring a *Candlelights* series—a series of inspirational books written *by* and *for* family caregivers, ministers, political leaders, medical students and a host of others of varying disciplines throughout the world.

Let us, as family caregivers, light nine candles to represent the nine virtues, namely: *Love, Joy, Peace, Patience, Kindness, Goodness, Faithfulness, Gentleness and Self-Control.* These nine virtues ("fruits of the spirit") will each be focused individually in the nine-book Candlelights series under the motif: *Transforming the World Through Deeds of Kindness, One Story at a Time.*

Life teaches us by human experiences that Kindness encompasses all of the virtues of praise without its vices and/or religious dogma. Kindness is the most graceful attitude you can assume toward another individual.

In gratitude for America's spirit of kindness and compassion that our nation has given and that family caregiving experiences have taught, we family caregivers of America can lift our lighted candles and shout from the depths of our hearts, "God Bless America, my home, sweet home!" And, in the words of Maltrie D. Babcock: "Be strong! We are not here to play to dream, to drift; we have hard work to do and loads to lift. Shun not the struggle, face it; 'tis God's gift. Be strong, be strong!"

Then, clutching our spiritual keys, we can answer President Bush's call to continue being strong and courageous in using our myriad of talents to build this great nation. We family caregivers can join his army of strength and courage by lifting high our lighted candles and begin our mission to help transform the world through deeds of *kindness*, one story at a time for the purpose of touching lives and lifting spirits.

On the spiritual journey, we can quote lyrics from the song, *Lead Kindly Light*, written by John Newman, and silently pray into the inherited *Eternal Light* of our awakened family caregivers' world.

2
Universal Candlelights for The World

Lead, kindly light, amid the encircling gloom...Lead thou me on; The night is dark, and I am far from home... Lead, thou me on; Keep Thou my feet, I do not ask to see; The distant scene; one step enough for me. —John Newman

In a prayerful effort to conclude this book with some comforting words that life has taught through experiences of long-term family caregiving, I used the spiritual keys to unlock wisdom gained through hours of meditations and gratitude journal writing as I wrote through the pain of the recent terrorist attacks. Even as I was writing in the midst of silent tears, the song "We Are Going Home" continued to resonate in the quietness of my soul.

Being a family caregiver who has experienced shock and pain, and learning that they are prerequisites for spiritual growth, I feel the need to share comforting thoughts and feelings with our readers.

It is no coincidence that the "Kindly Light" led me to a

timely article regarding kindness written by the Dalai Lama and circulating in e-mail worldwide. The message voiced my same philosophy I have been highlighting throughout all my writings, especially in the book entitled *We Create Our Own Happiness: What Family Caregivers Have Learned About Life for the New Millennium.*

The following are some comforting words we now pass on to the world that project the basic philosophy of our "Candlelights" series under the motif: *Kindness is the True Universal Religion...* a belief that many spiritual leaders aforementioned in Chapter Four of this book, also embrace. We have borrowed liberally from the Delai Lama's essay as his expressions very beautifully echo our own.

Of Spiritual Thoughts and Feelings

Comfort ye, comfort ye my people, saith your God.
Isaiah 40:1

The shocking and devastating events of September 11, 2001 cause every thinking individual to stop and meditate deeply about the purpose of life. Similar to the experiences of long-term family caregiving, we all search again for not only the meaning of life, but the purpose of our individual and collective experiences as we have created them—and we look earnestly for ways in which we might recreate ourselves as human beings, so that we will never treat each other this evil way again—the epitome of man's inhumanity to man.

The time has come for us to show, by human examples, our thoughts and feelings about Who We Really Are and Where Are We Going. Wisdom tells us that there are two possible responses to what has occurred on September 11, 2001. The first comes from the wisdom of **love**, the second from the attitude of **fear**. If we come from fear we may panic and do things— because of our religious faith, race or nationality as individuals, or as nations—that could only cause further damage. If we come from **love** we will find wisdom, refuge, kindness and strength, even as we provide them to others.

This is the moment of our universal spiritual ministry. The painful events have shown us that God speaks to us through human experiences, commanding us to love one another and awakening us to transcendent wisdom and universal compassion. We learn from the painful experiences of the Jews being slaughtered and the Africans being kidnapped and brutally enslaved, that greater than life is our **personal** relationship with God who commands us to love one another.

This is the time for spiritual teaching. What we teach at this time, through our every word and action right now, will remain as indelible lessons in the hearts and minds of those whose lives we touch and whose spirits we lift both now, and for years to come.

We will set the course for tomorrow, today, as we put forth our best efforts to respect the universal law of cause and effect. At this hour, in this moment, let us seek not to pinpoint blame, but to pinpoint cause. Unless we take this time to look at the cause of our experiences, we will never remove ourselves from the experiences it creates. Instead, we will forever live in fear of retribution from those individuals who feel aggrieved, alienated, and, likewise, seek retribution from them.

To many of us, the fundamental reasons are clear. We have not understood the most basic spiritual wisdom that life teaches. We have not learned the most basic human lessons. We have not remembered the most basic human truths. In short, we have not been listening to God that we should love one another and because we have not, we watch ourselves do ungodly, evil things to one another.

The message we hear from all sources of truth is clear: **We are all one**. We **are** our brother's keeper. **We are interrelated, interdependent and interconnected**. This is a message that life has repeatedly taught and the human race has largely and repeatedly ignored. Ignoring this truth is the only cause of hatred and war, and the way to remember is simple: **Love, (in) this and every moment**. Kindness, indeed, is love in action. "Love, ye, one another."

Let us ask ourselves the questions: If we could love even those who have attacked us, and seek to understand why they have done so, what then would be our response? Yet, if we meet rage with rage, attack with attack, fear with fear, negativity with negativity, what then will be the outcome?

These are the basic questions that are placed before the human race today. They are questions that we have failed to answer for thousands of years because we choose to continually ignore them. Failure to answer them now could eliminate the need to answer them at all. If we want the beauty of the world that we have co-created with God to be experienced by our children and our children's children, we will have to become spiritual activists right here, right now, and cause that to happen. We must choose to be a spiritual cause in the matter. We must choose to be candlelights for the world!

So, let us talk with Eternal God today. Let us as a world ask Eternal God for divine guidance, for transcendent wisdom, for counsel and advice, for insight, for strength and for inner peace. Let us ask Eternal God to help us, as a world, to promote social justice, universal peace and brotherly love. Let us ask Eternal God **on this day** to show us how to Show

Up in the world in a way that will cause the world itself to change, and join all those people around the world who are praying right now, adding our **LIGHT** to the **LIGHT** that dispels all fear and evil. This, indeed, is the challenge that is placed before every thinking individual today.

Today, let each of us ask ourselves the serious question: What can I do to preserve the beauty and the wonder of our world and to eliminate the anger and hatred—and the disparity that inevitably causes it—in that part of the world which I touch? Can I be a candlelight of kindness?

Please seek to answer the question today, with all the magnificence that is YOU. What can You do TODAY...(at) this very moment? A basic teaching in most spiritual traditions is: What you wish to experience, provide for another.

Look to see, now, what it is you wish to experience—in your own life, and in the world. Then see if there is another for whom you may be the source of that. If you wish to better understand experiences that seem incomprehensible, help another to better understand. If you wish to know that you are safe, cause others to know that they are safe. If you wish to experience peace, provide peace for another.

If we wish to walk with each other in perfect harmony and heal our own sadness or anger, we must seek to heal the sadness or anger of others. Those others who are "our brothers" are waiting for us now. They are looking to us for guidance, for help, for courage, for strength, for understanding, for wisdom and for assurance at this hour. Most of all, they are looking to us for love. Kindness is love in action.

The world needs kindness. Man will reach God only through his brother in deeds of kindness. The love of our brother is the essential action of human existence. The love of our brother is the only way in which we can experience God.

Yes, kindness is love in action. KINDNESS IS THE TRUE UNIVERSAL RELIGION! Kindness is the act of creation and the constant preservation of the world in existence. Kindness springs from the soul of man; it is the nobility of man—-a divine rather than a human being. From divine kindness flows, as from a fountain, the powers and the blessings of all created kindness. The power of kindness is not in what it does for us, but where it leads us: at once to the heart of humanity and therefore to God. We are awakened to the wisdom that all creation is holy, even our adversities.

God wants to enter the world in us and through us. He wants to be kind through us. Our disabled brothers teach us this powerful lesson daily through long-term family caregiving experiences. Through family caregiving experiences, our disabled brothers teach us that God is life, and to love one another is to see His face. As candlelights for the world, it is our spiritual mission to shine our light of kindness to help heal the world through deeds of love and mercy, and let our voices resonate from the depths of our hearts...

Lead on, O King Eternal, 'till sin's fierce war shall cease,
And holiness shall whisper the sweet amen of peace.
For not with swords' loud clashing, nor roll
of stirring drums, But deeds of love and mercy,
Thy heavenly kingdom comes.

Appendix

CAREGIVING TIPS FOR HELPING THE DISABLED AND/OR THOSE FACING A SERIOUS ILLNESS

We all are aware that when someone we know is ill or disabled, we often feel a sense of helplessness because we aren't sure of ways in which we can assist. Below are some caregiving tips that can be used to help in your mission of touching lives and lifting spirits.

WHEN I CRY FOR HELP...

1. Please don't avoid me. Be a dear friend...the loved one you've always been.

2. Touch me. A simple squeeze of my hand can tell me you still care.

3. Call me to tell me you're bringing my favorite dish and what time you're coming. Please bring food in disposable containers, so I won't need to worry about returns.

4. Help me feel good about myself. Tell me I look great, considering my illness.

5. Please include me in decision making. I've been robbed of so many things. Please don't deny me a chance to make a decision in my family...my life.

6. Talk to me of the future. Tomorrow, next week, next year. Hope is so important to me.

7. Please take care of my children for me. I need a little time to be alone with my spouse. My children may also need a little vacation from my illness.

8. Weep with me when I weep. Laugh with me when I laugh. Don't be afraid to share this with me.

9. Bring me a positive attitude. It's contagious!

10. What's in the news? Share magazines, photos, newspapers, verbal reports. Keep me from feeling the world is passing me by.

11. Take me out for a pleasure trip, but know my limitations.

12. Call for my shopping list and make a "special" delivery to my home.

13. Talk with me about the joy of being grateful.

14. Call me before you visit, but don't be afraid to visit. I need you. I am lonely.

15. Help me celebrate holidays (and life) by decorating my room or home or bringing me tiny gifts of flowers or other natural treasures.

16. Help my family. I am sick but they may be suffering. Offer to come stay with me to give my loved ones a break. Invite them out. Take them places.

17. Could you help me with some cleaning? During my illness my family and I still face dirty clothes, dirty dishes and a dirty house.

18. Be creative! Bring me a book of thoughts, taped music, a poster for my wall, cookies to share with my family and friends, or bring an old friend who hasn't come to visit me yet.

19. Let's talk about it. Maybe I need to talk about my illness. Find out by asking me: "Do you feel like talking about it?"

20. Don't always feel we have to talk. We can sit silently together.

21. Can you take me or my children somewhere? I may need transportation to a treatment...to the store...to a doctor.

22. Won't you please water my flowers?

23. Just send a card to say "I care!"

24. Pray for me and share your faith with me.

25. Tell me what you'd like to do for me and, when I agree, please do it!

26. Please tell me about support groups so I can share my thoughts and feelings with others who understand.

27. Please pray with me sometimes; and take me to church services sometimes.

28. Help me write some letters to my friends thanking them for their thoughtfulness.

29. Please read the Scriptures to me sometimes.

30. Please help me write my thoughts and feelings in my gratitude journal. I'll tell you what to write.

RESOURCES FOR THE CAREGIVER

Support Organizations and Newsletters

(1) National Family Caregivers Association, *Take Care: Self-Care for the Family Caregiver.* Kensington, Maryland. A Quarterly Newsletter.

The National Family Caregivers Association is a not-for-profit membership organization dedicated to improving the quality of life of America's 18,000,000 family caregivers.

Telephone: 301—942-6430/800-896-3650

Website: www.nfcacares.org Email: info@nfcacares.org

(2) *Today's Caregiver Magazine*, Hollywood, Florida.

Today's Caregiver Magazine is the best resource of information that addresses caregivers' needs and concerns. Every issue features an interview with a celebrity caregiver and a range of articles on topics such as incontinence, mobility, Alzheimer's caregiving, legal and insurance issues, nutrition and so much more.

Telephone: 954-893-0550. Fax: 954-893-1779 Outside Florida 800-829-2734

E-mail at editor@caregiver.com

Website: www.caregiver.com

(3) Well Spouse Foundation. *Mainstay: A Newsletter of Well Spouse Foundation.* New York, NY.

Well Spouse Foundation is a national non-profit organization formed to give emotional support, raise consciousness about, and advocate for the spouses and children of the chronically ill.

Telephone: 800-838-0879.

E-mail: wellspouse@aol.com

Website: www.wellspouse.org

BOOKS

Canfield, Jack, Mark Van Hansen and Bud Gardner, *Chicken Soup for the Writer's Soul*. Health Communications, Inc. Deerfield Beach, Florida, 2001.

Carroll, David, *Living with Dying: A Loving Guide for Family and Close Friends*, New York: Paragon House, rev., 1991.

Friedman, Jo-Ann, *Home Health Care: A Complete Guide for Patients and Their Families*. New York: W. W. Norton, 1986.

Hooyman, Nancy R., and Wendy Lustbader. Taking *Care of Your Aging Family Members: A Practical Guide.* New York: Free Press, 1986.

Johnson, Alice. *Caring for the Caregiver: A Manual for Those Who Care for Disabled Family Members or Friends*. Miami, Florida: Mal-Jonal Productions, Inc., 1998.

Rob, Caroline, R.N. *The Caregiver's Guide: Helping Elderly Relatives Cope with Health and Safety Problems*. Boston: Houghton Mifflin, 1991.

Rollin, Betty. *Last Wish*. New York: Warner, 1985.

Strong, Maggie. *Mainstay: For the Well Spouse of the Chronically Ill.* New York: Penguin Viking, 1988.

Van Brommel, Harry, *Choices for People Who Have a Terminal Illness and Their Families and Their Caregivers*. Toronto: NC Press Limited, 2nd Rev. ed.

Candle Lights

FOR THE WORLD

Transforming the World Through Deeds of Kindness

Guidelines for Writing "Candlelights" Stories for the Book Series

GUIDELINES

Dear Friend of our Candlelights Series,

In the international war against terrorism, it is great, artistic writers like you who can help transform the world through spiritual stories of kindness from your personal world of kind thoughts, feelings and actions. We all love reading about human experiences that touch lives and lift spirits, and it is our hope that you have a myriad of inspirational stories to share for our Candlelights series to help spread love throughout the world.

1. The Three Proponents of an Acceptable "Candlelights" Story

(1) A "Candlelights" story is a true, inspirational story about people courageously performing deeds of **kindness** for another person. It is a dramatic and emotional story that touches lives and lifts spirits, and that covers the range of human emotions. It is an inter-denominational, spiritual and human work of art that helps the readers discover basic, simple strategies they can use in their own worlds to promote inner peace and experience abundant life...spiritually, physically and financially.

(2) A "Candlelights" story has a unique beginning, middle and ending that closes with a moral and powerful pizzazz. It is a personal story that comes from the depths of the heart, enabling the reader to feel more grateful, compassionate and loving; more enlightened, awakened and alive with the spirit of kindness.

(3) A "Candlelights" story awakens the reader to our human interconnectedness, interrelatedness and interdependence, enabling her/him to joyfully feel as one in the heart of all creation.

2. Specific Guidelines for a "Candlelights" Story Portraying kindness

(1) Writing deeply from the heart and portraying the human experience, tell a true story about a courageous deed of kindness that was performed by you or someone you know. Remember to stay focused on your subject of kindness because Kindness is love in action.

(2) With a passion, write your true story in a dramatic way that will trigger a myriad of spiritual thoughts, feelings and actions. Let your story have literary value. Include dialogue.

(3) Let your story (a) begin with a problem, situation or issue. In other words, put your protagonist high up in a tree and throw darts at him/her, (2) let the problem, situation or issue include thoughts, feelings and actions, and (3) let it end with a result, such as a lesson learned, a transformed life, or a spiritual surprise.

Because kindness encompasses all the virtues, you may focus any one of the following nine virtues: (1) Love, (2) Joy, (3) Peace, (4) Patience, (5) Kindness, (6) Goodness, (7) Faithfulness, (8) Gentleness, and (9) Self-Control. Remember, you may write more than one story.

3. A "Candlelights" Story is Not: An autobiography, a eulogy, sermon, term paper, dissertation, personal testimony; a commentary on politics or controversial subjects.

4. How to Submit Your "Candlelights" Story

(1) Submit your story typed on plain white "8 1/2 X 11" paper, in 12-point Times New Roman font. Double spaced. 300-1200 words. Include a 25-50-word bio about you and/or about your latest book or project .

(2) We do not return submissions, so please do not send us your original copy.

(3) Unless you are writing for your assigned "Candlelights" series co-author of the book, you may submit your story to:

Mal-Jonal Productions, Inc.
Att: Alice W. Johnson, Ed.D.
Candlelights Series
16713 SW 107th Place
Miami, Florida, 33157-2965

5. About Your Published Story

Once we receive your story, we will mail you an acknowledgment card. If your story is published, you will be given a free copy of the book, and your name will be noted as author of the story. Proceeds from book sales will be awarded you through your specified organization, school, college or university department that solicited your story/stories and who will be the co-author of the book. Now is the time for you to be published and to help win the war against terrorism by sharing your stories of kindness to help transform the world. Kindness is the true, universal religion and your inherited divinity.

The Candlelights Series Editors
Mal-Jonal Productions, Inc., 16713 SW 107 Place,
Miami, FL 33157-2965
Tele: 305-253-4061 • Fax: 305-235-2600.
E-Mail: alicejohnsonmj@aol.com

Dear "Candlelights" Story Prospective Author,

The following are eleven "Candlelights" titles now underway for the first 9-set series. Each of the eleven (11) books will consist of nine chapters (the nine virtues of God) with 2001 words in each chapter. Thus we have the " 9/11/2001" that unified us as a spiritual world on September 11, 2001, a date we shall always remember with deep compassion. Each of the books have professional co-authors with a passion for creatively "Writing for Him" and spreading love to help transform the world through kindness.

(1) Candlelights for the Family Caregiver's World

Candlelights for the Family Caregiver's World is the first volume in the series, and is the spinoff for the rest of the books. It is a very different book from the others because it is not a collection of stories. Rather, it is a book written by a family caregiver that focuses six spiritual keys of wisdom for avoiding caregiver-burnout and promoting inner peace. The book shows why family caregiving is a spiritual mission that teaches us the wisdom of kindness toward others. Thus, we learn from the experiences of family caregiving that our disabled loved ones are here to teach us **the wisdom of kindness.**

The following ten titles are spinoffs of *Candlelights for the Family Caregiver's World.* Each book will consist of a collection of 110 short stories of 1492 to 2001 words based on the specific guidelines given. The stories will portray courageous acts of kindness. The number, "110," represents the "110" members of the United Nations, an organization of nations that work for international peace and security. The number "1492" will represent the year America was discovered , and "2001" will represent the year of the terrorists attacks. The stories will be a memorial to America's 9/11/2001 experience, shining candlelights of kindness into the thoughts, feelings and actions of humanity; transforming the world, one story at a time. The moral of each "Candlelights" story will be: "Touching Lives, Lifting Spirits."

(2) Candlelights for the Family Caregiver's World... Book #2 (Local/National)
(3) Candlelights for the The Family Caregiver's World...Book #3 (International)
(4) Candlelights for the High School Student's World
(5) Candlelights for the Medical Student's World
(6) Candlelights for the Clergyman's World
(7) Candlelights for the College Student's World
(8) Candlelights for the Mother's Spiritual World
(9) Candlelights for the Spiritual Teenager's World
(10) Candlelights for the Married Couple's World
(11) Candlelights for the Religions of the World (Through The National Organization of Church Women United)

"God Speaks to Our Hearts through Human Experiences"

Greater than life is our personal relationship with God, who commands us to love one another and who awakens us to transcendent wisdom and universal compassion.

This truth is beautifully exemplified in the following inspirational books written by writer/producers Alice Ward Johnson, Ed.D., and her chronically ill husband, John Johnson, Ed.D.

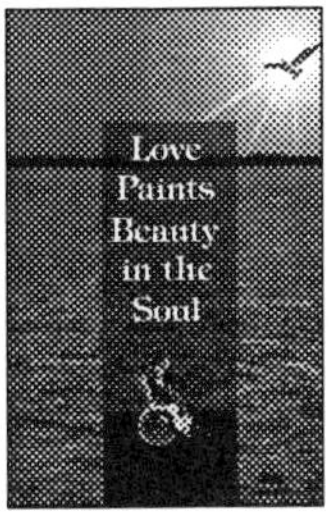

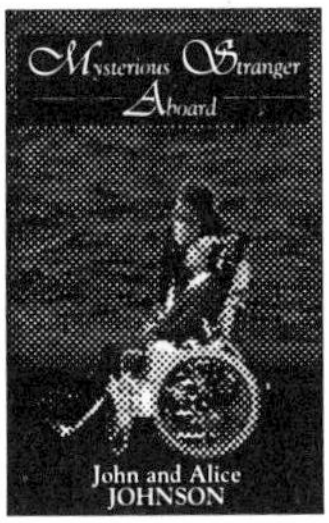

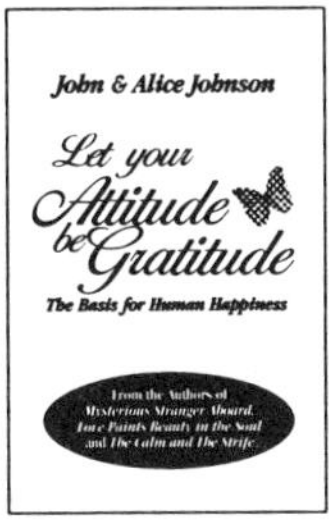

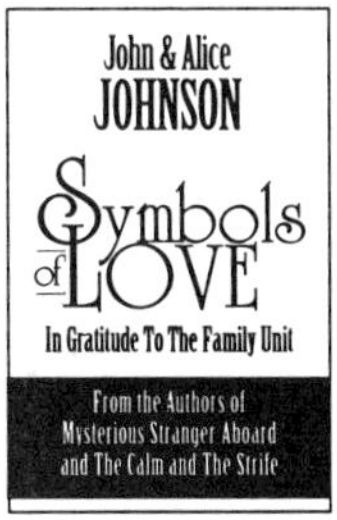

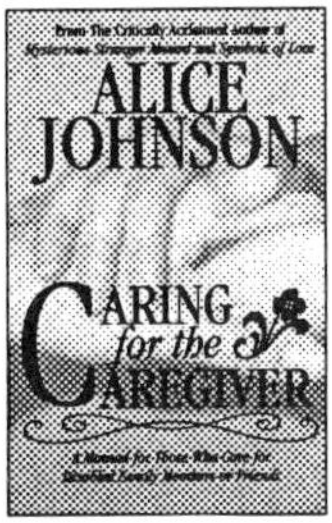

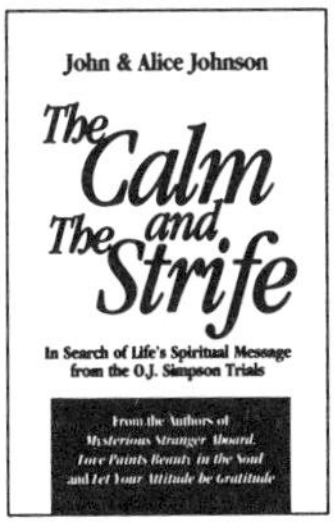

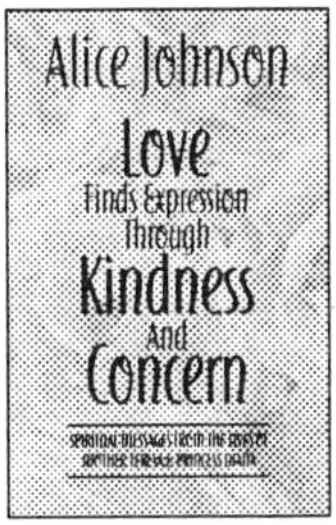

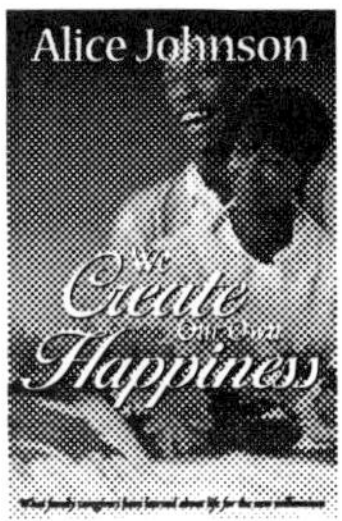

THESE ARE MUST-READ BOOKS BY THE JOHNSONS!

Mal-Jonal Productions, Inc.

16713 SW 107th Place • Miami, FL 33157
Phone # 305-253-4061 • Fax # 305-235-2600

ABOUT THE AUTHOR

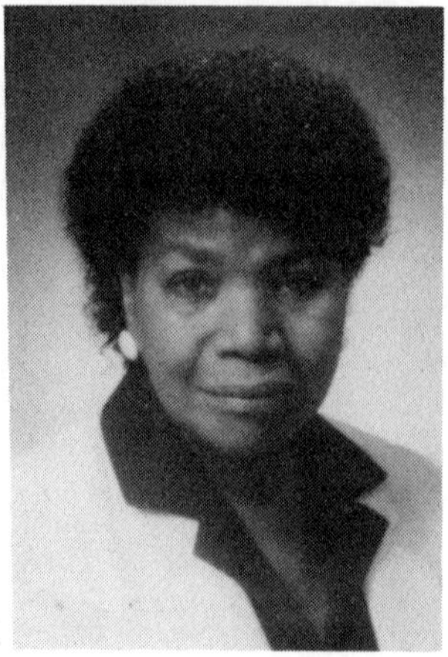

ALICE JOHNSON is a writer/producer and a graduate of Savannah State University and Clark-Atlanta University. She and husband John, a Morehouse College and University of Cincinnati graduate who is a victim of multiple sclerosis, have written nine books of inspiration, volumes of musical docudramas emphasizing multicultural education and literacy, and poetry portraying the human experience. The authors have been awarded numerous honors for their creative writings as caregiver and patient and their record is included in the 1999-2000 edition of *Marquis Who's Who in the South and Southwest*. Alice was honored with the *2000 Care Hero Award* presented by the national magazine *Today's Caregiver*.

ORDER FORM

BOOK TITLE	QUANTITY
~*Mysterious Stranger Aboard*	________
~*Love Paints Beauty in the Soul*	________
~*The Calm and The Strife*	________
~*Let your Attitude be Gratitude*	________
~*Symbols of Love*	________
~*Caring for the Caregiver*	________
~*Love Finds Expression through kindness and Concern*	________
~ *We Create Our Own Happiness*	________
~ *Candlelights for the Family Caregiver's World*	________

$10.00 EACH OR $5.00 EACH FOR ORDERS OF 20 OR MORE!

Name ____

Address ____

City/State/Zip ____

Phone Number ____________________ Fax Number ____________________

Make checks payable to Mal-Jonal Productions and mail to:
Mal-Jonal Productions, Inc.
16713 SW 107th Place
Miami, Florida 33157

sharing your stories of kindness to help transform the world. Kindness is the true, universal religion and your inherited divinity.

The Candlelights Series Editors
Mal-Jonal Productions, Inc., 16713 SW 107 Place,
Miami, FL 33157-2965
Tele: 305-253-4061 • Fax: 305-235-2600.
E-Mail: alicejohnsonmj@aol.com

Dear "Candlelights" Story Prospective Author,

The following are eleven "Candlelights" titles now underway for the first 9-set series. Each of the eleven (11) books will consist of nine chapters (the nine virtues of God) with 2001 words in each chapter. Thus we have the " 9/11/2001" that unified us as a spiritual world on September 11, 2001, a date we shall always remember with deep compassion. Each of the books have professional co-authors with a passion for creatively "Writing for Him" and spreading love to help transform the world through kindness.

(1) Candlelights for the Family Caregiver's World

Candlelights for the Family Caregiver's World is the first volume in the series, and is the spinoff for the rest of the books. It is a very different book from the others because it is not a collection of stories. Rather, it is a book written by a family caregiver that focuses six spiritual keys of wisdom for avoiding caregiver-burnout and promoting inner peace. The book shows why family caregiving is a spiritual mission that teaches us the wisdom of kindness toward others. Thus, we learn from the experiences of family caregiving that our disabled loved ones are here to teach us **the wisdom of kindness.**

The following ten titles are spinoffs of *Candlelights for the Family Caregiver's World.* Each book will consist of a collection of 110 short stories of 1492 to 2001 words based on the specific guidelines given. The stories will portray courageous acts of kindness. The number, "110," represents the "110" members of the United Nations, an organization of nations that work for international peace and security. The number "1492" will represent the year America was discovered , and "2001" will represent the year of the terrorists attacks. The stories will be a memorial to America's 9/11/2001 experience, shining candlelights of kindness into the thoughts, feelings and actions of humanity; transforming the world, one story at a time. The moral of each "Candlelights" story will be: "Touching Lives, Lifting Spirits."

(2) Candlelights for the Family Caregiver's World... Book #2 (Local/National)
(3) Candlelights for the The Family Caregiver's World...Book #3 (International)
(4) Candlelights for the High School Student's World
(5) Candlelights for the Medical Student's World
(6) Candlelights for the Clergyman's World
(7) Candlelights for the College Student's World
(8) Candlelights for the Mother's Spiritual World
(9) Candlelights for the Spiritual Teenager's World
(10) Candlelights for the Married Couple's World
(11) Candlelights for the Religions of the World (Through The National Organization of Church Women United)

"God Speaks to Our Hearts through Human Experiences"

Greater than life is our personal relationship with God, who commands us to love one another and who awakens us to transcendent wisdom and universal compassion.

This truth is beautifully exemplified in the following inspirational books written by writer/producers Alice Ward Johnson, Ed.D., and her chronically ill husband, John Johnson, Ed.D.

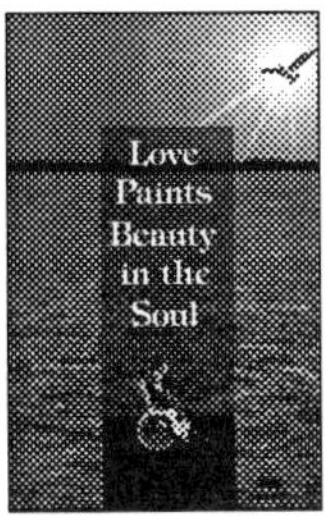

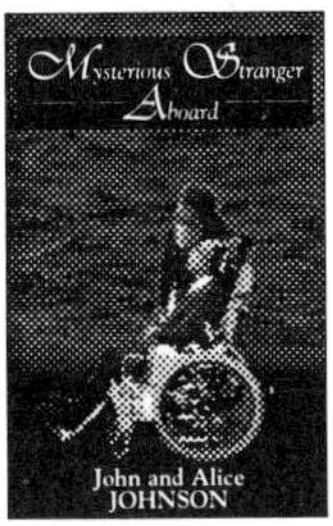

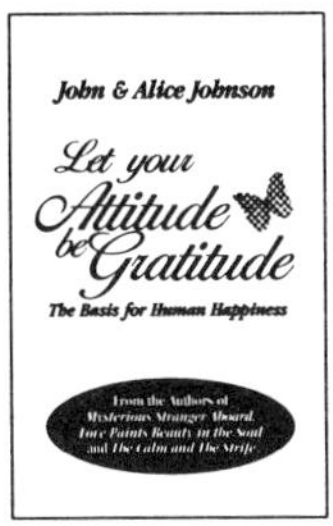

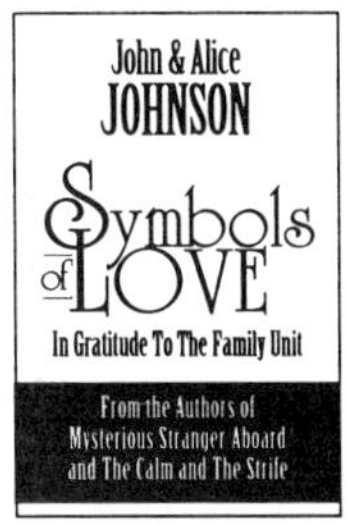

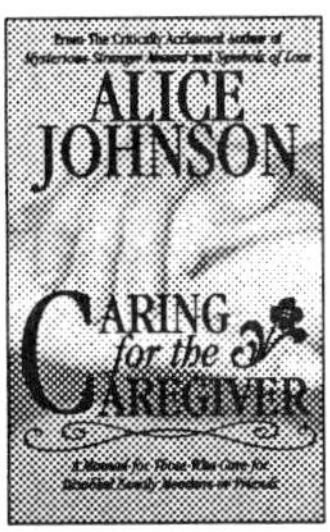

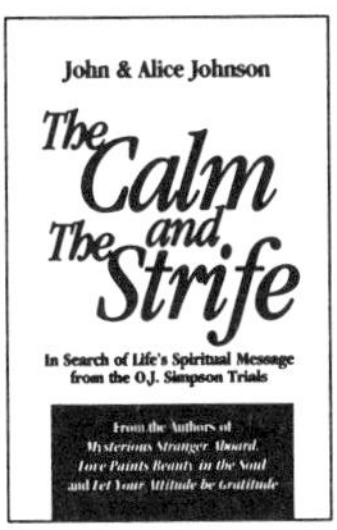

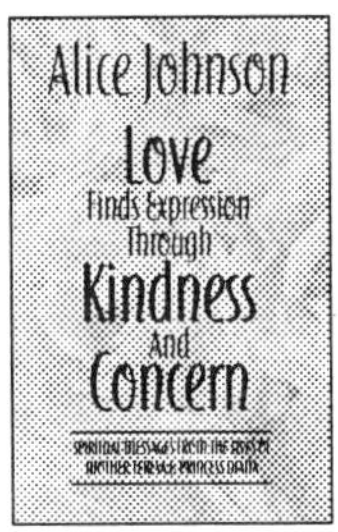

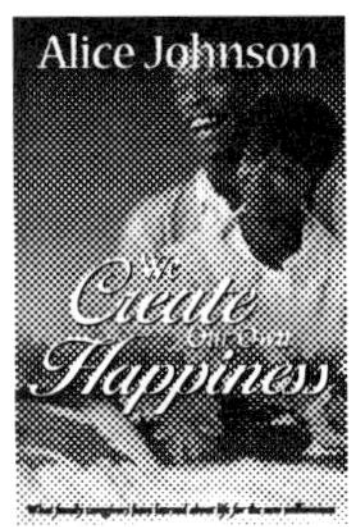

THESE ARE MUST-READ BOOKS BY THE JOHNSONS!

Mal-Jonal Productions, Inc.

16713 SW 107th Place • Miami, FL 33157

Phone # 305-253-4061 • Fax # 305-235-2600

ABOUT THE AUTHOR

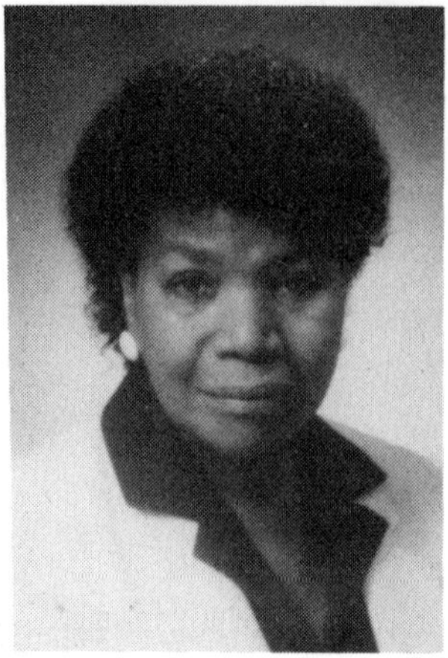

ALICE JOHNSON is a writer/producer and a graduate of Savannah State University and Clark-Atlanta University. She and husband John, a Morehouse College and University of Cincinnati graduate who is a victim of multiple sclerosis, have written nine books of inspiration, volumes of musical docudramas emphasizing multicultural education and literacy, and poetry portraying the human experience. The authors have been awarded numerous honors for their creative writings as caregiver and patient and their record is included in the 1999-2000 edition of *Marquis Who's Who in the South and Southwest*. Alice was honored with the *2000 Care Hero Award* presented by the national magazine *Today's Caregiver*.

ORDER FORM

BOOK TITLE	QUANTITY
~*Mysterious Stranger Aboard*	________
~*Love Paints Beauty in the Soul*	________
~*The Calm and The Strife*	________
~*Let your Attitude be Gratitude*	________
~*Symbols of Love*	________
~*Caring for the Caregiver*	________
~*Love Finds Expression through kindness and Concern*	________
~ *We Create Our Own Happiness*	________
~ *Candlelights for the Family Caregiver's World*	________

$10.00 EACH OR $5.00 EACH FOR ORDERS OF 20 OR MORE!

Name ______________________________

Address ______________________________

City/State/Zip ______________________________

Phone Number ______________ Fax Number ______________

Make checks payable to Mal-Jonal Productions and mail to:

Mal-Jonal Productions, Inc.

16713 SW 107th Place

Miami, Florida 33157